Keeping Your Smile

⋰⋱

OTHER REDLEAF PRESS BOOKS BY JEFF A. JOHNSON

Babies in the Rain: Promoting Play, Exploration, and Discovery with Infants and Toddlers (2010)

Everyday Early Learning: Easy and Fun Activities and Toys Made from Stuff You Can Find Around the House (2008) by Jeff A. Johnson with Zoë Johnson

Finding Your Smile Again: A Child Care Professional's Guide to Reducing Stress and Avoiding Burnout (2007)

Do-It-Yourself Early Learning: Fun Activities and Toys from Everyday Home Center Materials (2006) by Jeff A. Johnson and Tasha A. Johnson

❦ ❦ ❦

Keeping Your Smile

Caring for Children with Joy, Love, and Intention

JEFF A. JOHNSON

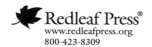

Redleaf Press®
www.redleafpress.org
800-423-8309

Published by Redleaf Press
10 Yorkton Court
St. Paul, MN 55117
www.redleafpress.org

First edition 2010
Cover design by Elizabeth Berry
Interior design by Jim Handrigan and typeset in Stempel Schneidler and Meta
Printed in the United States of America
18 17 16 15 14 13 12 11   2 3 4 5 6 7 8 9

Library of Congress Cataloging-in-Publication Data

Johnson, Jeff A., 1969–
    Keeping your smile : caring for children with joy, love, and intention /
Jeff A. Johnson.
       p. cm.
    ISBN 978-1-933653-85-3 (alk. paper)
    1. Child care workers—Psychology. 2. Child care services—Psychological
aspects. 3. Burn out (Psychology)   I. Title.
HQ778.5.J64 2010
362.701'9—dc22
                              2009039498

Printed on acid-free paper

In memory of Chris Blades, who provided the tools
I needed to keep my smile and taught me to let go.

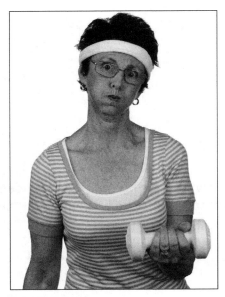

All things are difficult before they are easy.

—*Thomas Fuller,* Gnomologia: Adages and Proverbs

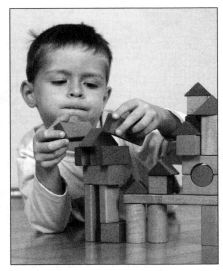

Nothing in the world is difficult for one who sets his mind to it.

—*Anonymous*

Contents

Foreword

I'VE BEEN A WIFE SINCE 1972, a mother since 1973, and a tutu (that's Hawaiian for grandmother) since 1997. I have spent most of my adult life working directly with children as a family child care provider or working as an advocate for other professional caregivers. I was the CEO of my family child care business for eighteen and a half years and I enjoyed every minute of it—almost. Even during the beginning years when I was simply a "babysitter" I felt a sense of purpose. I did many things the hard way over the years, but I was always growing. Sometimes the growth was slow—it wasn't until six years after opening my "babysitting service" that someone coached me to find my path as a child care professional. I soon found this was my real passion and I've never stopped smiling. There have been good times and bad times, there have been times of flow and times of struggle, there have been times of sickness and times of health, but through it all I still have my smile and there are plenty of people smiling back at me.

Many of you are like me, managing to navigate a course through life that leads to some sort of passion or purpose. We know where we are going, but there are plenty of bumps and some wrong turns along the way. Others may be leading lives full of motion, but lacking focus, direction, and lasting happiness. You may be feeling "stuck" or "lost in your own life." Whether you are on the path to living what Jeff calls your

Ultimate Purpose, or still trying to determine exactly what your purpose is, this book is for you.

In my opinion, Jeff wrote this book to help us all "check in" with ourselves and make sure we find and stay on our personal paths—wherever those paths may lead. Life is a once in a life-time adventure, and we should be smiling and having fun as we make our way through it. We don't get to start over or go back to that place where we think we made a mistake for a "do over." We never get to take back bad choices, angry words, nasty looks, or self-neglect.

In *Keeping Your Smile,* Jeff helps us to realize that we have to be mindful of our choices and find time in our hectic days to take a deep breath now and then. We have to make sure we are taking care of ourselves and not neglecting to meet our own needs. Throughout the book, he encourages

- making it okay to put ourselves first now and then;
- focusing on and work to live our goals and dreams;
- looking at our follies and missteps and learning from them;
- exploring how our past influences our present and future;
- dusting off the cobwebs of our lives to find our smile;
- thinking positively and looking for good in every situation;
- taking chances and moving out of our comfort zones;
- living with passion and purpose.

Jeff also encourages us to deal with the tough parts of life most of us prefer to ignore. The truth is that keeping your smile requires dealing with your dark secrets and dirty laundry. Jeff asks us to do some real soul searching in this book, but he does it gently—with humor, wit, and irreverence—which makes look-ing deep into the corners of your mind a bit easier. This book is a toolbox full of helpful questions, activities, and practices that you can dig into and use to find what you need to live a joyous and solidly happy life. It will help you not only keep your smile, but also keep it forever polished and shiny. Jeff has provided the tools, but you have to take action and use them.

Jeff is a person who makes anyone around him for any length of time smile, and this book reflects that. He can't help himself; he is a happy soul, and he wants everyone in his world to be happy too. In this book, Jeff does what I expected him to do; he shares his smile, wit, and honest passion for the welfare of children across this nation. You see, this book was ultimately written for our children. While it is full of tools and support for caregivers, at its core it is a guide for providing high quality care to children and creating nurturing learning environments.

I first met Jeff via e-mail and telephone back in 2003 when he and his wife, Tasha, were transitioning from a center-based child care program to their own family child care program. He was looking for information and support on how to "do" quality family child care. I helped him find resources and knew from the beginning that they were right on track. I could tell the children in their care would be on a wonderful roller coaster ride of HAPPY, because Jeff and Tasha had learned to put themselves first. They had learned to take care of their own needs, and this meant they were grounded and better able to take care of the needs of the children in their care. The mind-set of adults working with children is very important. Caregivers who radiate happiness and joy teach children to smile and to keep smiling. They make kids who are fearful feel secure in this great big world. They help children become self-reliant and productive. And most importantly, they are better able to tune in to the unique needs of individual children. This book is Jeff's way of providing our children what they need: caregivers who continue to smile at work and play; people like you and me who are passionate about our "jobs" as child care providers, parents, grandparents, and teachers. This is a one-size-fits-all book, written for anyone who works with, or cares for, young children.

Jeff is committed to children of all sizes, even the children still inside of us grownups. In this book, he offers up tools caregivers who are mildly frustrated, worn out, stressed, off course, or lost can use to stay on (or find) their path. You are in for a treat, because this wonderful book will help you "check in" on yourself. When Jeff sent me the *Keeping Your Smile* manuscript, I read it and completed the activities (be sure to have a pen or pencil handy while reading this book!). I felt very happy and was totally smiling when I finished because I know I am truly living my "Ultimate Purpose."

Hang on and enjoy the rollercoaster ride that is your life. Keeping your smile through all the ups and downs takes commitment, but it is well worth the time and effort you invest. Reading this delightful book helps remind you to live *your* life to its fullest and to live for *your* dreams and ideals, not the dreams and ideals of others. When you are content and fully living your life, you will give off positive vibes that help those around you. When you smile real smiles at the world, the world smiles back.

Aloha!

—Daphne Naleilehuaokaala Cole
TOPSTAR, Tennessee's Family Child Care
Peer Mentoring Program Director

Acknowledgments

THANKS TO TASHA, MY WIFE, my one true love, and the reason for most of my smiles. Your support makes everything I do possible. Thanks for taking such good care of me.

Thanks to the thousands of caregivers and parents I have talked to over the last few years. Your stories about how your smiles shine and fade are the foundation for this book.

Thanks to my editor, Beth Wallace, for nudging me along and honing my thinking through the creation of this book. Thanks to Laura Maki, Jim Handrigan, JoAnne Voltz, and Linda Hein at Redleaf Press, who had hands in the production, design, marketing, and publishing of this book, and special thanks to David Heath and Kyra Ostendorf for all the support they provided.

Thanks to the country of Ireland. Your beautiful countryside, stunning seashores, and inviting pubs made revising this book a joy. Special thanks to Billy at the Anchor Bar in Courtmacsherry. The incredible live music and friendliness at the Anchor in the evenings and the wonderful outings you suggested for the day-light hours made settling down and working on this book much easier.

Introduction

I'M A FAMILY CHILD CARE PROVIDER and proud of it. Before that I was the director of a center-based child care program, a job that made me equally proud. For over twenty years I have watched and helped children of all ages discover bits and pieces of their world. I have seen a lot of firsts: first children, first steps, first words, first friendships, first laughs, first encounters with mud, first fights, first skinned knees, first falls from an apple tree, first baskets from the free throw line, first days of school, first tastes of spinach, first report cards, first words written and read, first jumps from the side of a pool, first trips to the zoo, first home runs, and first slivers in frightened children's fingers.

All of these things bring a smile to my face. They are the reasons I go to work every morning. Supporting, nurturing, guiding, and sometimes nudging children as they develop brings meaning to my life.

I know I am not alone. Over the years, I have met thousands of parents, child care providers, foster parents, grandparents, and teachers who believe working with children is more than a job. They believe it is a calling. They believe it is their Ultimate Purpose in life, the reason for their smile.

This is understandable, because so many of us approach our jobs from a position of hope, joy, love, and happiness. We throw ourselves into our work too. We work until we are exhausted.

Then we work a little more. Then we sleep for a while. Then we get up and do it all over again the next day.

The mistake too many caregivers make is that they get so busy taking care of others that they fail to care for themselves. If you are happy and love your work, you owe it to yourself to take care of your own needs so you can continue to be happy and love your work. If you feel stress slithering into your life a bit more than you would like, you need to take action before it takes over.

We love our work so much that it often means tolerating pitiful work conditions, benefits, and pay. It also means physically and emotionally draining work that often goes unnoticed, long hours that are unappreciated, and self-sacrifice that is unacknowledged. We know deep in our heads and hearts we are doing good, but most of us long to hear someone say, "Thank you!" and to receive some recognition for our commitment to children and families.

While most caregivers are appreciated and valued, it is not verbalized frequently enough. Children are usually too young to recognize and appreciate their caregivers' good works, and parents often are so caught up in their own hectic lives that they don't think to voice their gratitude.

This was on my mind when I received an e-mail from a parent explaining that her caregiver was "truly a godsend." She explained that her child care provider was not only great with her children but had done a lot to help her become a better parent.

In my reply, I asked if she wouldn't mind sharing how this provider had been a positive influence. She agreed to let me share it here. I've changed some details and names to protect her privacy.

> I married at twenty-one and had two children in the marriage. I was young and made some poor choices and stayed in a failing, scary marriage "for my kids" until they were four and one-and-a-half. When I left, I basically snuck out with the boys and what I could fit in a backpack and came home to the Midwest. I went back to college, stayed single, and got a good job.

At this point, her two boys started child care in the home of the provider who turned out to be a "godsend." I will call her

Jane. Her boys thrived in the program and eventually outgrew it when they started school.

Later, I became engaged to a man I worked with and saw roses in my future! I became pregnant a couple months before the wedding; we were planning on me being able to stay at home with the baby, as I had always wanted! Six weeks before the wedding, my fiancé committed suicide.

Dealing with suicide is hard. Being pregnant and not married at that point in my life was tough. I was ashamed of myself. I was thinking I should have seen something only God knew. Jane agreed to watch the baby if I needed her to.

Her baby girl started in Jane's program when mom went back to work. At four months of age, she was diagnosed with food allergies. She was nursing and allergic to things her mommy was eating. Mom changed her eating habits.

When the baby was about seven months old, Jane and I knew something was not right. That is such a hard thing to face when it's your kid. She was not sitting up independently, not swallowing like she should, and she would cry and scream. Finally, Jane took my hands, looked me in the eyes, and showed me the developmental chart she has on her fridge.

Jane told me what my daughter should be doing at this age and that I should get her a developmental evaluation. Jane said if she was wrong that was okay. She loved us too much to see something and not say anything.

The baby was evaluated and they found she had significant physical delays, but no mental delays. The food allergies were depriving her of nutrients. The nutrients she got went to her brain and eyes, causing small and large muscle delays.

She is now working with speech, physical, and occupational therapists. All of the therapy is done at Jane's house, so I don't have to take off work. At each progress meeting, I hear accolades for Jane by the therapists. Many of them comment on how much they wish all the families they work with had such good support by everyone who interacts with the kids. The baby is still behind and hanging on to the bottom of the growth chart, but making progress. She is on a new medicine that has been wonderful!

Jeff, I have thanked God so many times that Jane had the courage to speak up. I was in such denial. I was so afraid it would be something so bad. I was paralyzed. We are fortunate. In a few years, God willing, you will never know she was behind.

I believe care providers are in a unique position that allows them to really see these kids around their peers and compare them objectively. It must have taken a lot of courage for Jane to tell me she thought there was a problem, and I am glad she did!

I could go on and on with stories of our time with Jane in the last eight years. I will just say I thank God for her. She is a wonderful friend and has allowed me to go to work without worrying about the care my kids get. Many single moms I know have had their careers suffer because of unreliable child care, and I am fortunate to have never known what that is like. I am fortunate to have someone in my life like Jane who stuck with me through all of this.

I know Jane. She has a positive impact on the children and families in her National Association for Family Child Care (NAFCC) accredited program, and it goes further. She is a leader in her state and a role model to child care professionals beyond her state's borders. She lives hundreds of miles from me but has influenced my own growth as a professional. She is strong, direct, energetic, and fun and is always thinking about how to make things a little better. She also takes care of her own needs; she maintains her smile so it is always burning bright.

Imagine for a moment what the story might have been like if Jane had lost her ever-present smile. Imagine her weighed down by stress. Imagine her unhappy in her career choice and bogged down by life. She might have opted not to take this family into her program. She might not have been tuned-in enough to notice the infant's delays. She might not have felt compelled to say anything if she had noticed. She might not have had the energy to advocate for quality care in her state and beyond.

Luckily for many of us, Jane takes care of herself. She manages her stress well. She knows when to say "no." She understands her own limitations. The smile and positive energy she puts out into the world comes back to her again and again.

If you are a caregiver—a parent, a child care provider, a teacher, a foster parent—who feels called to do the work you do, if you feel caregiving is your Ultimate Purpose on this earth, if you are driven to make life better for children and families, I am sure you are someone's Jane.

You may not always feel appreciated; you may not hear the words of thanks your ears ache for; you may not always think the effort is worth the payoff, but make no mistake about it, you are someone's godsend—and that is why your smile matters.

Strong Smile or Frustrated Frown?

It is sad that so many people responsible for creating environments for children that are pro-learning, pro-love, pro-hope, pro-joy, pro-success, pro-growth, pro-happiness, and pro-thought feel stuck in their own lives, drained of their passion, and hopelessly adrift. Life overwhelms them. Once strong and resilient smiles wilt into tense grimaces or frustrated frowns.

Do any of these things sound familiar?

- While things are usually okay, there are moments now and then when you feel overwhelmed by life.
- Sometimes you feel like parts of your life just are not "clicking," that they are out of sync.
- Your mental chatter becomes so loud and overpowering that it interferes with your ability to focus on what is going on in your life right now, in this moment.
- At times you feel little or no control over what is happening in your life.
- You want to make life-improving changes, but can't find the time, energy, or inspiration to take action.
- You dread things in your life that formerly brought joy to your day and made you smile.

- You frequently wear a happy-face mask for the world to hide discomfort and unhappiness.

Caring for children is both physically and emotionally demanding work that tends to consume caregivers. So much time, energy, and other resources go into nurturing the children in your life that there is nothing left to nurture your own needs. Caregivers such as you habitually relegate personal needs to the bottom of too long to-do lists. Time never seems abundant enough to do what needs doing. Important activities are put off until later, and time to pursue dreams and personal ambitions doesn't seem to exist.

No matter how busy you are, don't let your to-do list consume your smile. Doing so starts you down a road away from your dreams and passions and inspirations. Your smile is important because it is an indicator of your inner state. Think about how you feel in your head and heart when you

- smile sarcastically at someone who is irritating you;
- smile fully and for real at your sweetie;
- can't even force a phony smile for someone who usually makes your smile shine;
- smile and laugh deeply until your sides hurt;
- fake a smile because it is expected of you.

Take some time to think about your relationship with your smile:

- Does your smile come easily or is its appearance rare?
- Was your most recent smile real or was it a show for the people around you?
- Do you feel your life lacks smiles or overflows with them?

Recently Annie, a bright-eyed two-year-old who has been in our family child care program since she was a newborn, walked up to me smiling ear to ear. One-year-old Brenden was right behind her babbling and smiling. Annie's right arm was outstretched, and she was gently holding something between her little thumb and index finger. She wore an "I have something special for you" look on her face.

I realized holding out my hand was a mistake as I saw a large, dry, greenish booger falling from her fingers as she said, "I got it out. It's Brenden's." I smiled a huge and very real smile as I thanked her.

There have been times in my life when my reaction would have been different, times when I could not muster a smile for such a gift, times when I probably would have snapped at her for picking her friend's nose, times when I could not see the humor in the image of Brenden standing tolerantly while Annie dug in his nose. When you are two, you can pick your friends, you can pick your nose, *and* you can pick your friend's nose.

Life is full of smile-sharing opportunities, but hectic lives blind us to many of them. When life is over and you are about to take your last breath, do you think you'll wish for time to check more items off your never ending to-do list or time to honestly smile at little friends sharing large, dry, greenish boogers?

Have You Seen a Lost Smile?

I directed a child care center and community center for sixteen years. My wife Tasha worked as my assistant for most of that time. She had known she was burning out for years. I had no idea it was happening to me until one day in early 2003 when I blew up and quit my job. Our smiles were lost. We put on happy faces for work and then went home and barely spoke. A few years later, I looked back on that time in our life and commented to Tasha that staying in those jobs two more years would have killed our marriage. She replied, "It would not have taken that long."

This book grew out of my lost smile. The transition from empty and smile-less to fulfilled and smiling was long and hard, but more importantly, it was avoidable. My hope is that this book helps you manage your stress, keep your smile, and maintain an abundance of joy, love, and intentionality.

Keeping Your Smile is intended for adults who want to keep their heads and hearts in the right place while caring for children. Family and center-based child care providers, parents, teachers, foster parents, and grandparents will benefit from what follows. When the term "caregiver" is used it is intended to refer to all of the above groups. If you wish to keep smiling while doing right by young children, this book is for you.

Can You Take Control?

At its heart, this book is about taking active control of your life so you can maintain your smile. What *control* looks like in your life is as unique as you are. For some readers, control means being more aware of the choices. For others, it means learning to relax and investing time in self-renewal. Some may find it means making changes to the way they act and interact as they go about their days. Some could see a need for small modifications in their routines, while others will decide they need to make major changes. Some might realize taking control means changing careers or making other life-altering transformations.

My hope is that this book helps you see options and make healthier choices for keeping your smile. This book should help you

- take control of things in your life you need to be on top of and let the rest go;
- stay fully engaged in your life;
- grow and change in the ways that best serve you and your purpose in life;
- name and meet your unique needs;
- simplify;
- know your Ultimate Purpose and let it guide your choices;
- dance through the highs and lows of life with a hopeful smile.

Want to Know What's Ahead?

The first three chapters look at the things that steal our smiles and cause all that distracting background noise that clouds our thinking. These chapters also look at the physical, emotional, spiritual, and psychological costs of fading smiles. The next five chapters look at ways to regain control of your life and offer tools for dealing with your unique adversities. The final chapter wraps things up and empowers you to get up and do the work necessary to keep your smile.

Taking care of yourself can be daunting. You get so busy taking care of everyone else that you forget to care for yourself, or you are just too exhausted at the end of the day, or you feel guilty taking care of yourself when that time could be spent caring for someone else, or you just don't feel like there is enough time in the day to carve out 10 minutes just for you. To make things a bit easier, the staff at Explorations Early Learning LLC have developed a few inventions that are described in boxed sections throughout the book to help you on your quest for a balanced and fulfilling life. Keep your eye out for these inventions. We really think they will help bring back your smile!

Can We Make a Connection?

Authors piece together words, sentences, paragraphs, and chapters based on their unique life experience, knowledge, and accumulated opinions. Then readers bring *their* personal life experience, knowledge, and accumulated opinions with them as they read. As a writer, my goal is to build a bridge between what I bring to the book and what you bring. Our experiences separate us, so do time and space. I am sitting at my kitchen table here in Iowa typing these words into my laptop a few days before Christmas 2008. The first draft of the manuscript will be finished in six months, then it goes through developmental editing, a revision, substantive editing, more revision, copy editing, and layout and design before printing and shipping. You are reading this long after I wrote it and are probably not sitting at my kitchen table. (If you *are* at my kitchen table, give me a wave when I walk by and ask me to bring you a cup of coffee or a glass of wine.)

Another thing separating me as an author from most of the people reading this book is my gender. The vast majority of readers are women, and I have to do my best to speak to you. That means trying to use complete sentences instead of grunts and hand gestures. I also try not to refer to spitting, scratching, belching, and other stereotypical male misbehavior too often. (Although I have met some female child care professionals over the last few years who are first class spitters and belchers. As a gentleman, I will not name them here.)

These differences in experience, time, space, and gender make interaction between you and me challenging. I want you to feel I am talking directly to you, but the unique and personal things about ourselves that we bring to the book means I'm not always going to get it right. I also want to make the book as interactive as possible, another challenge of time and space. As an author, I want to make as strong a connection with you as possible, but in the end, I am more concerned about empowering you to connect with yourself. As you read, I want you to relax and bring as much of your true self to this book as possible. That might mean thinking about things you usually don't think about and letting go of things you work hard to control. It might not be easy, but you can do it. In the end, it leads to a stronger smile.

Ready to Giterdun?

Reading is pretty passive. You sit, and you read. Sure, you make some mental connections with the text, but the process is pretty still. Reading does not burn many calories. To encourage interaction, this book is full of questions and opportunities for action. I urge you to take time for them. You'll get more from the text if you take your time and participate. We live in a rush-through-this-to-get-to-that-and-then-go-on-to-the-next-thing world. It does you good to pause and look inside your head now and again. Locating ideas, feelings, and opinions you may have misplaced or forgotten is good for you. To make it easy, I have left plenty of space or provided lines for you to answer questions, jot notes, and scribble ideas. I want you to feel like we are interacting, but another goal is to create some interaction between you and your inner self. I have a vision of your copy of my book dog-eared, written-in, highlighted, and worn from use, sitting within easy reach while you are out living life with a huge smile on your face.

A few notes about the questions and activities to come:

- They are meant to tap into your experience, knowledge, and dreams and help you to clarify your thinking and feelings.
- There is no wrong way to do an activity or answer a question. There is no test. There are no grades. You get an A+ just for picking up your pen and writing.

- Another goal of the questions and activities is to urge you to act on your own behalf. Maintaining your smile is an active process and requires action.

Scribbling answers to all the questions and doing all the activities will not burn many more calories than just reading, but it will burn a few. More importantly, it will take you further down the road toward keeping your smile than simply zipping through the text.

Can You Commit to Following Through?

Years ago, I bought a book about canoeing. I had never been canoeing before, but it looked like fun. I wanted to buy a canoe and learn how to handle it in the water. Reading the book gave me lots of good advice and tips: wear a life vest, practice on a calm lake your first time out, make sure your canoe is securely tied to the vehicle on the way to the water. The book offered practical and simple recommendations about canoeing, but it was not canoeing. To really canoe, I had to put down the book, get my canoe wet, and start paddling. You do not learn how to canoe by reading about canoeing; you learn how to canoe by canoeing.

The differences were vast. I was not scared of tipping over while reading, and my shoes did not get wet while reading. The sensory experience was hugely different. Reading made canoeing *sound* fun; actually canoeing *was* fun.

Likewise, this book gives you some good information, but it does not help you keep your smile. Maintaining your smile requires action and hard work from you. The best this book can do is provide insight, offer ideas, and share tools. Keeping your smile takes commitment and effort on your part; no one can do it for you. You have to put your paddle in the water.

What Happens When You're Done Reading?

Action and change are up to you, but I wanted to offer support beyond the pages of this book. With that in mind, I have created for you on my Web site some Internet-based support intended to help keep your smile:

- The Explorations Early Learning Enews is an electronic newsletter containing articles and resources that goes to thousands of caregivers and parents around the world each month. Subscribe at www.explorationsearlylearning .com.

- The Explorations Early Learning Facebook page is a place where you can ask questions, get answers, and vent frustrations. Click "like" to join the discussion.

- The Keeping Your Smile blog is meant to help remind you to take care of yourself and maintain your smile. The short posts won't take up a lot of your time, but they do remind you to take a few moments each day for yourself. Check it out at http://keepingyoursmile.blogspot.com. You can even subscribe and have postings delivered directly to your inbox.

It is my hope that these tools help you make needed changes in your life, help you maintain your focus, and help you keep your smile for the long haul. Now, take a few long deep breaths, let your mind settle, and we'll begin.

One

Butterflies
and Barbed Wire

Your home is not your own, and it is not easy being a wife, mother, and childminder. It is not easy keeping on top of housework, and the necessary paperwork for your business, and then opening the door with a smile.

—*Marilyn Farlow*

DEEP BREATHING IS HELPFUL because it can create calm when life is most cluttered and hectic. Cleansing breaths help encourage calm and create space between you and whatever is stressing you out. Sometimes life is overwhelmingly complicated and in your face. Big and little stressors build until you feel like you are walking around with butterflies and barbed wire in your belly. Your neck and shoulders ache. Your head throbs. Your chest tightens. You feel empty or lost or about to burst or spent or exhausted or apathetic or ungrounded or edgy or adrift or *underwater* or like you just can't take *it* anymore. Sometimes you might even start thinking about trees.

"I knew I was losing my smile when I started thinking about the trees."

After I give a talk about stress and burnout, I ask caregivers and parents to share their stories and experiences.

"I saw them every morning in a big, inviting clump along the road as I drove to work."

The people sharing these stories often feel their smile fading and know it influences the quality of their interactions with children and the quality of their life in general. They frequently use words such as the ones that follow to describe the combination of barbed wire and butterflies swirling around their gut and head:

stressed	fearful	drained
anxious	tired	panicky
empty	broken	nervous
exhausted	scared	gloomy
miserable	scarred	jumpy
hollow	depressed	sad

"I tried to calculate in my head . . ."

Some feel they relinquished control of their lives at some point along the way and desperately want to take it back. The tunnel vision that burnout brings leaves them feeling their options are limited. They are so overwhelmed by the situation that they cannot see the world of choices available to them.

". . . how hard would I have to hit them . . ."

Instead of seeing a world of options, their minds focus like lasers on the stress and tension eating away at them. Their singular focus overshadows dreams and goals, clutters emotions, drains joyfulness, and kills relationships.

". . . to hurt myself enough to get some rest in the hospital but not quite kill myself."

Minds are often consumed with hurtful and dangerous thoughts meant to stop suffering and resuscitate dying smiles.

"I thought it was the only way I would be able to find some calm and clear my head."

The first time a provider said she had contemplated driving into a clump of trees so she could get some rest and maybe get her smile back for a while during rehab, I was worried. When I heard an almost identical story from another provider a thousand miles away, I was shocked. Hearing a third version of the story from yet another caregiver was numbing. These same stories were not just a coincidence. They revealed the reality that the job of a caregiver can eat away at one's happiness—for even the most dedicated caregiver—if that caregiver does not make a conscious effort to maintain his or her happiness.

You are almost certainly not thinking about driving into a clump of trees. In fact, you probably still enjoy your job (at least most of the time) and love the challenges, the smiling faces, and the busy little brains. It is a lot of work, and you're good at it. You feel confident and capable most of the time. Some days, though, things get stressful, leaving you tense and overwhelmed. When this happens, you usually bounce back quickly. Overall, you're probably happy and content most of the time.

It is important that you manage your stress so you do not get to the point where it consumes you. The three women who shared stories about their thoughts of harming themselves used to be in your position. They loved their jobs. They were dedicated and passionate about their work. Then, gradually, there were more bad days and bouncing back was tougher. As time passed, they started feeling like they had less control over their lives. Eventually, those dark thoughts started to pop into their heads. You have to take conscious control of your own well-being right now so this slow, downward spiral does not happen to you.

This book is one of the best tools you have for understanding why your smile fades and for making mindful changes to help maintain your smile. If you skip over the questions and activities presented here, you are cheating yourself and missing opportunities to better understand yourself and your situation in life. You might think you don't have time to stop, think, and write. You might feel doing these things won't do you any good. You might be scared you'll open emotional wounds and think about things that you work very hard not to think about. You made a financial investment when you purchased this book, and you have invested time in reading so far. Why not invest a bit more time and a little energy in answering the questions you could just skip past? The worst that could happen is you spend time alone inside your head thinking about things you need to think about. I think you are worth the effort.

What's Your *It?*

Even when you are having a great day, a day when noses are not running, no one has been bitten, and everyone slept well the night before, something can pop up and throw things off. I don't know what your *it* is, but sometimes *it* gets to you. This chapter is about your *it* or, more likely, your *its*—those things that get under your skin and cause your pulse to quicken, your breathing to shorten, and your smile to fade. Your *it* might be

- lack of appreciation for your work;
- the way a particular child's voice rubs against your delicate last nerve;
- long working hours;
- life whooshing by;
- a pile of unending paperwork;
- something painful you've carried for years or decades.

We will get to some common stress causers and smile stealers in a bit, but first I want you to take time to identify and know some of your *its* a tad better. Take a few moments to clear your head and find some calm.

1. Start with a few long, deep breaths, fully emptying and fully filling your lungs.
2. Exhale until your lungs feel like they have collapsed.
3. Inhale until you cannot possibly inhale any more.
4. Pause at the top and bottom of each breath.
5. Repeat.
6. Continue until you find an inner stillness.

Now, pick up your pen and answer the following questions:

What three sights, sounds, or experiences cause your smile to fade?

_____

_____

_____

What happens in your body when you are under stress? What happens in your mind?

_____

_____

_____

How do you react to stress? What do you do or fail to do? How do you behave with other people?

_____

_____

_____

Take a few more long and deep cleansing breaths. Close your eyes and on the inside of your eyelids create an image of you and the thing that stresses you the most. In the space provided, draw the image you just created. You do not have to be an artist to do this; just do your best to put the mental image on paper. It sounds silly, but taking time to recreate this mental image makes _it_ more real and helps you better understand your relationship with your stress.

What Are the Signs?

While we all suffer from our *its* in unique and special ways, their impact on our bodies, attitudes, and outlooks is similar. The following are some common signs that your *its* are overwhelming you and leading you away from your smile and toward burnout. If stress and burnout don't have much hold on you, you may only experience symptoms occasionally—on those rare days when your *it* attacks. You probably don't experience more than a few of them, and they don't hit you that hard. On the other hand, if your stress and burnout are stronger, multiple symptoms may be a part of your daily life, and those symptoms may be nearly overwhelming. You may even start thinking about driving into a clump of trees.

HEADACHES AND MUSCLE TENSION

It may be a sharp pain in the center of your head, as if someone just jammed a freshly sharpened number two pencil through your left ear into your brain. It may be a numbness that throbs through your whole head, although for the life of you there is no memory of being injected with 60 cc of Novocain. Then again, it may not be your head. It could be your shoulders that ache like they are carrying the weight of the world or a neck so stiff you can't look both ways before crossing the street or a lower back that won't bend or knees and feet that burn with pain. Physical discomfort is an early sign of stress for many people.

PHYSICAL AND EMOTIONAL AILMENTS

The physical signs of stress can go deeper than headaches and muscle pain. Over the last few years, I have met many providers and parents stressed to the point of physical and emotional illness. One family child care provider said that after repeated tests failed to diagnose the reason for an ongoing problem, her doctor asked her a simple question, "Are you experiencing any stress in your life?" Since this was the first time she remembered being asked this question, she answered "yes" and then spent half an hour providing details. His diagnosis was quick and simple: "If you don't deal with it all, it could kill you." Researchers are continuing to find connections between stress and illness that back up this anecdotal evidence. In my own experience, I have found I am healthier when I manage my stress effectively. My body simply works better when I invest time in the things that work for me, things such as yoga, meditation, running, reading, and woodworking.

INSOMNIA

Raise your hand if you have trouble sleeping. When I ask groups of parents and caregivers to do this, 75 percent of them raise their hands. As we discuss the topic, they explain that their days are so full they do not have time for all the sleep they need, and when they do finally settle into bed, their minds are cluttered with thoughts and worries about yesterday and tomorrow. The mental chatter makes sleep difficult and uneasy.

ABSENTEEISM OR PERFORMANCE DECLINE

When the stress starts getting to us, we tend to stop showing up for the things that cause the stress, or when we do show up, we "phone it in," just go through the motions. (This may explain why I skipped so many days during my senior year of high school!) Center directors can predict when staff members are going to quit by tracking how often they call in sick on Fridays and Mondays. Why would you want to show up at a place that is making you physically ill and affecting your sleep? Why would you want to pour any more of yourself into work that is causing you so much stress?

IRRITABILITY AND INCREASED ANXIETY

When you are not sleeping, when your body is aching, and when you are feeling ill, there is a good chance you might be a tad irritable or anxious. You begin to snip and snap at the people around you, your pet becomes afraid of you, your chest tightens, and you end up feeling fed up and scared of the world.

BOREDOM, APATHY, AND DEPRESSION

As burnout builds, you may find yourself apathetic and bored with life. The day-to-day sameness of your home life and job leave you feeling bored and unfulfilled. You struggle to keep up appearances, but something is missing. You find it hard to care as much, or as deeply, as you once did about your work. As time goes by, you realize that you've been down so long that it's hard to remember up. You feel depressed. That feeling may be fleeting or it may hang on like a nit to a strand of hair. If your feelings of depression are ongoing, it is important that you reach out for the help you need. There is nothing wrong with asking for help when you need it.

ESCAPE ACTIVITIES

At times the feelings of stress and anxiety build to the point where you need to take the edge off in order to function at all. There are times when you simply need to escape from your *its*. Methods of escape vary for each of us. Maybe you take the edge off with chocolate, wine, or exercise. Maybe you need to veg out with a few hours of *Law and Order* reruns a few nights a week. Maybe cruising the Internet helps to clear your head. Maybe five minutes alone in the bathroom without someone twisting the doorknob and asking, "whatchadoin? whatchadoin? whatchadoin?" is your idea of escape. As stress builds, we begin to feel empty, and escape activities are a quick way to put gas into our tanks.

ADDICTIONS

Chronically stressed people often rely so heavily on their favorite escape activity that it becomes an addiction. A few pieces of chocolate now and then can turn into an eating disorder; drinks after work once in a while can turn into alcoholism; buying a sexy pair of shoes every few weeks can turn into an uncontrollable urge to shop. Escaping from your stress feels good and you want to feel good all the time, which can end up in your losing control over your life.

TENSIONS WITH FAMILY AND FRIENDS

The tension with family and friends that Tasha and I experienced while we were burning out was incredibly painful and numbing. It's sad, but the more stress and burnout increase, the more we isolate ourselves from the important people around us. The people we should be reaching out to for help are the ones we push away, blame for our discomfort, and heap our anger on. Failing to deal with stress kills relationships and ends marriages. It drives an emotional wedge between you and people you care about. It presses so heavily on you that you lash out, ignore, or disrespect the individuals you love most. If it's hard for you to think about making time to manage your stress, here's something to think about: how do you think your stress is affecting the children in your care and the people you love? If it's hard for you to take care of yourself for your own sake, it may be easier if at first you do it for others, for the people who count on you.

☹ ☺ ☺

We are now going to work on better identifying the things that take our smiles, because understanding those things is the first step toward controlling them.

PERSONAL GPS

Your Personal Goal Positioning System (GPS) helps you stay focused on achieving your personal goals. Hectic lives blow too many people off course and away from achieving their goals. The hand-held Personal GPS lets you know at a glance on its touch screen where you are in relation to a variety of your long- and short-term goals. Its soothing audio directions even help guide you toward attaining goals you may feel are unreachable.

The system relies on your Emotional Positioning System, a series of high orbit satellites designed to track your emotional state, as well as neural sensors that transmit your goals and intentions to a central computer bank, located in a high security bunker off I-70 in central Missouri. With this system, you will never wake up in the middle of the night again wondering how you got so far off track from your dreams.

Ever Been Attacked by Snoterpillars?

Wild snoterpillars are a big annoyance for many caregivers, and they surely weaken my smile. At certain times of the year they run rampant through homes, schools, and child care programs around the country. It seems that as soon as you capture and dispose of one, another appears in its place. They just keep coming and coming and coming—they are unrelenting. They are a scourge on polite society.

Don't know what snoterpillars are? You've probably seen them and just did not know what to call them. They are those thick, usually green, caterpillar-like streams of snot that ooze from small children's noses.

I can't stand snoterpillars. Dealing with them and all the other things that leak, plop, spray, drip, or squirt out of children drive me crazy. They get under my skin and saw away at my nerves. They bring me to my knees. I cower when they attack, crouching in the corner with my hands over my eyes. I openly weep as Tasha scolds me, "Be a man. Just get a tissue and wipe it up before it gets all over the place." They are small; they are no real big deal; they come with the job; but they are also gooey and sticky and just plain gross. Snoterpillars are my kryptonite.

Bodily fluids don't bother everyone, but everyone is bothered by something. What are your snoterpillars? Knowing your snoterpillars, understanding their power over you, contemplating how they affect you, and thinking about why they affect you are big steps toward taking away their power. Bringing them from the darkness of your stressed-out mind into the light of day is empowering. The things that stress us out are often deeply personal and wholly unique. We all have different temperaments, tolerances, and breaking points. Right now, for example, I am sitting in a Nashville hotel writing while a few floors below me construction workers are chipping tile from a bathroom wall. The sound of their hammering is echoing through the ductwork, creating an almost rhythmic thump, thump . . . thumpthump. I'm typing through it, mostly unfazed. Tasha, on the other hand, escaped long ago. I could feel her annoyance growing as she tried to live with it, first reading, then adjusting the TV volume, and then covering her head with a pillow.

We all have different things that cause us stress to different degrees and for different reasons. We could broadly generalize about universal buttons caregivers share, but I think it is more important that you focus on knowing your buttons. These questions will help you find your snoterpillars:

What are some of the little things in your life that get under your skin?

_____

_____

_____

What happens in your body when you have to cope with these snoterpillars? What happens in your mind?

_____

_____

_____

How do you deal with them?

_____

_____

_____

Buttons, Buttons, Who Can Push My Buttons?

Certain people in my life were profoundly adept at pushing my buttons until I learned not to allow them that control. Sometimes their button pushing was intentional. When my daughter Zoë was little she would dramatically stomp to her room and slam the door when she was upset. It drove me up the wall, and she knew it. Her button pushing was intended to get back at me for whatever I had done to upset her. I'm sure she was thinking, "How dare you tell me to clean my room. I'll teach you!" as she stomp, stomp, stomped to her room and finished it off with a SLAM of the door. Others pushed my buttons unintentionally and probably unknowingly: the woman applying eye shadow while driving down the interstate at eighty miles an hour, the old lady in the express lane slowly writing a check for a single can of cat food, the father pushing his able-bodied four-year-old around the mall in a stroller, politicians (all of them). All these people pushed my buttons and flipped my smile into a scowl.

I'm not only a former victim of button pushing, I am also a card carrying member of the button pushers club. I know just the right words, body language, tones, and actions to touch, push, or slam the buttons of my wife, children, mother, siblings, friends, enemies, and acquaintances. I also must admit to pouncing on their buttons for reasons ranging from revenge to mischief to my own entertainment. I wish I was above such things. I wish I was more evolved. But not only have I pushed a lot of people's buttons in my day, I found it easy and took great joy in it. It felt good to make others miserable when I was feeling bad.

Life would be much easier if we were not all guilty of the same behaviors that drive us crazy when we see them in other people. I can't be too upset that Zoë pushed my buttons—she learned it from me. Let's dig down and see what you know about your buttons: Make a list of the people who push your buttons. Next to each name, list the button(s) they push. Simply being consciously aware of who pushes which buttons gives you more control over your life:

Do you know why they do so?

_____

_____

_____

_____

_____

_____

When are you more susceptible to having your buttons pushed? What makes you vulnerable at these times?

_____

_____

_____

Whose buttons do you take pleasure in pushing? What benefits do you get from pushing those buttons?

_____

_____

_____

Why are your buttons so sensitive? What makes you react so strongly to certain behaviors in other people?

_____

_____

_____

If I Close My Eyes, Will *It* Go Away?

Our buttons and the people who push them often become overwhelming and leave us wishing we could close our eyes and cast them away long enough to create a bit of calm, a bit of stillness, a bit of peace. The truth is you can find calm, stillness, and peace while closing your eyes, but you cannot keep your smile and deal with your stress by wishing away or hiding from your troubles. (Later in the book, I write about the tools of visualization and meditation, which are simple methods for clearing out mental clutter and bringing some stillness to your busy mind.) If your stress is not taking control of your life and if having your buttons pushed is only a minor irritant, you should consider yourself lucky. But you should also remember that not managing these things can lead to bigger problems down the road. *Now* is the time to make thoughtful changes. Taking control is a lot easier when you are not thinking about the clump of pine trees you pass on the way to work. You can learn to clear your mind, but when your eyes open all the things that stress you out are still waiting. As hard as I try to wish away snoterpillars when they attack, they are always hanging there waiting for me to deal with them when I open my eyes.

The emotional drain, snoterpillars, repetition, isolation, and other things that cause stress will always be around, but that does not mean these things must have power over your life. Some adults have felt powerless their whole life, others abdicated power along life's journey. Either way, this powerlessness you may feel in your own life can be overcome. You can be in control.

Your *intention* is an important player here. Before taking any action in your life, you must first think about it—intentions precede actions. You are reading this sentence because you picked up the book with the intention of reading. The intention, "I want to eat pizza" precedes the call to the pizzeria, which precedes the arrival of the pizza.

Our mind-set and outlook help determine our actions and reactions in the real world. What we put out into the world comes back to us, which means that putting a stressed, agitated, sad, fearful, or empty vibe out into the world brings those same things back to us. This creates a cycle of negativity that is hard to escape. As we move forward, I want you to consider what would happen in your life if you committed to taking a little more control of your life and focusing a little more on your own care. You can't always control your physical environment, but you do have control over how you react to that environment. As we delve in later chapters into altering our outlooks, I want you to have an open mind about changing your mind. For now, spend some time contemplating these questions:

What if you intended to live a life where you were in active control?

_____

_____

_____

What if your outlook shifted from seeing the negative in the world to seeing hope and opportunity?

_____

_____

_____

What if you put a positive vibe out into the world?

_____

_____

_____

Tactics, Tools, and Tips

1. Deep breathing is a valuable tool during life's most stressful moments. It clears your head, creates space between you and your situation, and helps you think better. The problem is that most people breathe shallowly, only using the top part of their lungs. Train yourself to breathe deeper by paying attention to how you inhale and exhale. Start by setting your cell phone timer or watch to beep every hour during the day. Then take five or six long, slow breaths every time you hear it. Make an effort to take some big breaths every time you feel the butterflies and barbed wire of stress. With time, you will train yourself to breathe better.

2. Review the answers, thoughts, and opinions you wrote down in this chapter. Now spend some time sitting with the feelings generated by those responses. We are usually in such a rush to move on to the next thing in our lives that we fail to spend time understanding and contemplating what we are feeling in any given moment. Sitting with your feelings, just spending time experiencing them, is healthier than ignoring them or suppressing them. Make sitting and communing with your feelings a new habit. When you feel stressed, happy, hurt, joyful, overwhelmed, or optimistic, pause for a moment to feel those things consciously. Become aware of

the physiological and emotional sensations they generate. Instead of running from your feelings, invest time in *knowing* them.

3. Earlier in this chapter you were asked to list the three *its* that cause the most stress in your life and to list some of the little things that get under your skin. What I would like you to do now is start a list of all the things in your life, big and small, that cause you stress. You may not have the time or mind-set to make a complete list all at once. That's okay. Just fold the corner of this page and come back to it as you think of things to add to your list. Knowing what gets to you—your *its*—is empowering; it gives you control and weakens the hold those things have on you. This detailed inventory of what causes your stress will be helpful later as you continue working to keep your smile. Plenty of space follows for you to make your list as comprehensive as possible.

_____

_____

_____

_____

_____

_____

_____

_____

_____

_____

_____

_____

_____

Two
Physical and Emotional Expenditures

CAREGIVERS EXPEND LOTS OF TIME, energy, and resources meeting the needs of children in their lives. This physically and emotionally demanding work is an undertaking that seems at times to have no end. The need for fresh diapers, healthy food, cuddle time, hugs, story books, role models, Band-Aids, tissue, naps, baths, eye contact, focused attention, discipline, humor, and so many, many more things is ongoing and unrelenting. Children are high-maintenance, ego-centric, self-absorbed, frequently smelly, sometimes intolerable, often loud bundles of curiosity, hope, joy, adventure, love, and silliness. The reason they are so darn cute is that if they weren't there is no way we could bring ourselves to tolerate them. The big bright eyes, ready love, and easy smiles are not just endearing—they are meant to manipulate us. For every annoyance, there is a bit of joy; for every crying fit, there is a quiet moment of cuddling; for every 3:36 AM feeding, there is a contented burp as they drift to sleep.

Many adults physically and emotionally break themselves for the well-being of the children in their care. Over the years, I've lost sleep; twisted ankles playing tag; stepped on Legos in bare feet; been kicked, head-butted, and punched in the groin; messed up my back lifting children; had my eyes poked and almost gouged out by curious toddler-fingers; and been scratched by razor-sharp infant fingernails. I've had to wait to pee until my bladder nearly burst; I've been peed on by infant boys and girls (on purpose?); I've felt the gentle spray of toddler sneezes showering my face; I've wiped up gallons of snot, buckets of puke, and pails of drool; and (believe it or not) I've even had to take a few sick days to fight the bacteria- and virus-borne illnesses kids have so readily shared.

The physical demands are great, but the emotional expenditures are probably more draining. It takes lots of empathy and compassion to create an emotional environment that consistently supports the needs of small children, and maintaining such an environment can suck the energy right out of you.

The emotional drain does not stop when children leave your care. Because you have put so much into them, the connections you formed last sometimes for years. As they grow up and move on, we rejoice when they succeed in school, get married, and live enjoyable lives. I love when "my" kids grow up happy, healthy, and fulfilled. I love knowing that way back when I helped lay the foundation for their success. We also mourn when they make bad choices, feeling like we failed to guide them in the right direction. I hate seeing adults who were once kids I worked with in the news for doing dumb, dangerous, or deadly things.

The strong connections and emotional bonds we build with children also leave us devastated when bad things happen to them later in life. I spent weeks in a funk after hearing that two young girls who once attended our family child care program were molested by a new caregiver. Tasha and I terminated care because the parents were unreliable and more challenging to work with than we wanted to tolerate. This was a hard decision because we had invested lots of time and energy in the girls, but it was the right thing to do for our own mental well-being. Hearing that some bastard put those girls through hell after I abandoned them due to their annoying parents shattered my heart. If I had sucked it up and tolerated the parents, the girls' pain would have never occurred. I ended up second guessing my decision, my commitment to children, and my generally positive world view. Then I took a deep breath, brushed myself off, and got back to work. A harsh reality of life is that bad stuff sometimes happens to innocent people.

We work until we're physically and emotionally exhausted. Then we work a little more. Then we blame ourselves for not doing more, or we question the quality of our work. And then? Well, then we wonder why we are suffering from the symptoms of burnout discussed in the previous chapter. We fail to connect our emotional exhaustion and physical aches and pains to the hard, draining work we do on behalf of those cuddly little kids. This is a cycle you must understand and learn to work with if you are going to keep your smile. Before we move on, here are three points I want you to remember:

1. Caregiving is physically and emotionally demanding.
2. Meeting those demands builds strong, lasting emotional ties with children.
3. Those demands can weigh on us, causing stress and dimming our smiles.

THE DO OVER

We've all been there before. A friend asks your opinion about whether a new boyfriend is as good as he seems, and you tell her what you *really* think. Before you have a chance to make up an acceptable lie, you inadvertently end up agreeing to coach a team of three- and four-year-old soccer players because you are known to be "good with kids." You carelessly gobble a whole quart of chunky chocolate brownie swirl ice cream after work instead of taking the long walk you had been planning all day. These things happen.

Wouldn't it be nice if you could go back and do these things over, making different decisions? Well, now you can. The Do Over is like a DVR for your life. Pushing the rewind button allows you to go back in time up to twenty-four hours to make better choices. With the Do Over, you can also

- fast forward through traffic or conversations with that annoying friend you don't want to be friends with anymore;
- push Pause to catch your breath during stressful moments;
- choose Slow Motion to make special moments last longer;
- replay events either because they were enjoyable or to make sure before you react that your goofy cousin Lenny said what you thought he said.

The Do Over will be available in three fashionable styles by the end of 2010 and is expected to retail for $329.95.

Why Don't You Go to Work?

I work long, hard hours and commit lots of physical and mental energy to my work, but I am frequently asked by preschoolers in our program things like, "Jeff, why don't you ever work?" "When are you going to get a job?" and "Why do you just play with us and read to us all day?"

Children have no idea how much work caring for them can be. I want to respond to their questions with something like: "Do you have any idea how many times I changed your diapers in the three years it took for you to learn to use the toilet? Do you know how hard it was to get you to nap when you were teething? Can you comprehend how much effort it takes to get your snot and drool off the windows and mirrors and how my spirit sinks knowing they only stay clean for an hour or so? Remember when you tried to flush your stuffed bunny? Do you not think cleaning up after the great flood was work? Oh, and what about the sand and dirt and everything else you track into the house? And the way you can turn your eyelids inside out to annoy me? And how you sneak up beside me and stick your wet finger in my ear when I am busy feeding a baby? Do you really think dealing with all of those things is not work?"

Instead of ranting and raving, I smile and say something like, "My job is to make sure you enjoy being a kid. How am I doing?" Then I smile inside and out because I know that part of doing my job well is to make it seem effortless to the children. If they don't think I am working, then I must be doing a good job of managing the physical and emotional expenditures that come with the job. Truth be told, I do not feel like what I do is work. I don't feel like I have worked a day since we started doing family child care in 2003. I'm often tired at the end of the day, but I am still smiling and eager for what comes next.

The job I burned-out at and left was work. It drained me. It sucked the life from me. It left me exhausted and empty at the end of the day. I often dreaded the coming day. I often felt emotionally shattered.

Here are some questions to consider before we move on:

What three things about your job are the most physically draining?

_____

_____

_____

What three things about your job are the most emotionally draining?

_____

_____

_____

What three emotions come to mind when you think about your job?

_____

_____

_____

When do you feel charged-up and excited about the work you do?

_____

_____

_____

How do you greet new workdays—with dread, or with anticipation? Why?

_____

_____

_____

Complete the following sentences:

When I think about my work, I feel . . .

_____

_____

_____

The thing I love the most about my job is . . .

_____

_____

_____

My biggest challenge at my job is . . .

_____

_____

_____

The thing about my job that most needs changing is . . .

_____

_____

_____

What's that Sucking Sound?

At first you might not hear it because it is not that obvious. After some time it builds and rings in your ears every time you exert yourself physically or emotionally for the children in your care. Then the sound becomes ever-present. You get to the point where you don't hear it unless something blasts it into your consciousness. It has become part of the background noise of your life. It is the sound of your exertions sucking time, energy, and resources right out of your life. On their own, your exertions as a caregiver don't make much noise, but when taken together, all the physical and emotional expenditures add up. You give and give and give and then give some more until you feel an all-consuming emptiness when you allow yourself to think about it.

The expenditures of time, energy, and resources are a necessary part of caregiving, but feeling that all-consuming emptiness is not. There are alternatives to the empty, smile-draining feelings, but they are hard to see when cocooned in comfortable layers of your own stress. The next chapters provide tools to help you see those alternatives and break free of your comfortable cocoon. For now, however, let's try to figure out more about how you expend your time, energy, and resources as a caregiver.

What Are the Costs of Caregiving?

When we think about the cost of caring for children, we probably think first about the financial expenditures: diapers, wipes, formula, jars of food, boxes of cereal, paper towels, toys, clothes, strollers, car seats, books, crayons, construction paper, shoes, Band-Aids, bigger clothes, bigger shoes, and on and on it goes. Children are constantly in need of some this or that—and even when a need is not readily noticeable, we often look for an excuse to buy, buy, buy. There is also a lot of pressure on parents and professional caregivers to succumb to social, peer, and media pressure to purchase stuff. I mean, what kind of parent are you if you do not spend $150 on the latest toddler running shoes or $1,500 on a Marc Jacobs stroller? How will Junior show his little face at the sandbox?

Kids are financially expensive, but the costs I want you to spend some time looking at are not monetary. For example, if you smoke two packs a day for twenty years, you have not only paid cash money for each cigarette; you have paid a physical price as well. The coughing, overtaxed heart, yellowed teeth, increased risk of cancer, exile to out of the way smoking areas, dirty looks from pious strangers, and shortened life span are some of the nonmonetary costs of your habit. The price you pay for those smokes is a lot more than the over the counter cost.

Before you can figure out how to keep your smile, you need to better understand the forces trying to take it away. With this in mind, I want you to spend some time looking at the nonmonetary costs of caregiving.

PHYSICAL COSTS OF CAREGIVING

Take some time to make a detailed list of the physical exertions that are part of your work with children during a given week—all the heavy lifting, bending, twisting, turning, chasing, cuddling, climbing, tumbling, stooping, wiping, scrubbing, dancing, running, hefting, hauling, pushing, and pulling you do. You might not be able to make this list all at once from memory. You probably do so much through habit that you don't even realize you are doing it all. That's okay. Just fold the corner of this page and try to be mindful of the physical work of caregiving you do over the next few days. When you "catch" yourself doing something physical, jot it down in the space provided.

_____

_____

_____

_____

_____

_____

_____

_____

Now look back on your list and make a star next to the activities you find draining, the ones that take the most out of you or cause the most wear and tear on your body. While you're reviewing the list, underline the items you enjoy, the ones that feel exhilarating or add a bounce to your step. This annotated list gives you an idea of all the hard physical work you do as a caregiver, and helps you identify the parts of the job you find most challenging and unpleasant.

EMOTIONAL COSTS OF CAREGIVING

It's not easy to list all the physical efforts that go into caring for a child, and listing all the emotional efforts is even more challenging. It's far easier to catch yourself wiping a nose or lifting a child than it is to catch yourself feeling any particular fleeting emotion. For one thing, emotions often move so fast that we barely notice one before another takes over our consciousness. We can go from happy to sad to aggravated and back to happy in a few moments, especially in a room full of hyperemotional children who are all just learning to experience and identify their own emotions.

Another problem with identifying the emotional cost of caregiving is the tendency to suppress, ignore, and fake our feelings. I used to think this was a guy thing, but after working in the predominately female early learning profession for over twenty years and meeting thousands of women, I now know better. It's not a guy thing; it's a human thing. Most of us are just not good at identifying our feelings. We don't know what to make of them. We find ourselves faking emotions we enjoy and would like to feel more often (pretending to be content, or happy, or fulfilled) and we run from the "bad" emotions like anger, fear, and sorrow (pretending that we don't feel them by stuffing them inside and ignoring them). This is tragic because the core of quality caregiving is the formation of strong emotional environments that are safe, nurturing, loving, and relaxed, and we do not do a very good job building these environments when we are hiding from our own true feelings.

WHAT'S THAT FEELING?

Most of us didn't grow up with help identifying our complicated feelings. "Glad," "mad," "happy," or "sad" might be the best we can do at first. Some folks even have trouble getting beyond "good" and "bad." To help you out, here's a list of basic feelings we all experience at one time or another:

afraid	disappointed	lonely
amazed	discouraged	nervous
amused	eager	optimistic
angry	embarrassed	overwhelmed
annoyed	exasperated	peaceful
anxious	excited	pleased
apathetic	frustrated	proud
bored	glad	puzzled
calm	grateful	rebellious
cheerful	helpless	relieved
comfortable	hopeful	reluctant
concerned	hopeless	sad
confident	hurt	surprised
confused	impatient	touched
curious	inspired	troubled
delighted	joyous	trusting

So, this might be hard for you, but I want you to create two lists over the next three days. The first is a list of all the things you catch yourself feeling in that time period. Make an effort to be emotionally self-aware. Think about how you are feeling. Then write down the feelings you experience. If you feel something more than once, just add a tally mark next to it on your list. For example, a portion of your list might look like this:

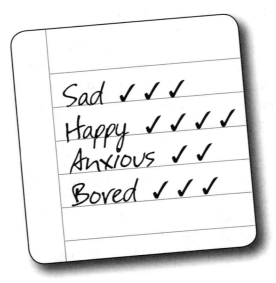

This list gives you an idea about your feelings as well as what you are feeling most. Creating it also helps you become more mindful about and aware of your feelings. You may sometimes feel confused, because naming your feelings is not always easy!

My Feelings

_____

_____

_____

_____

_____

_____

_____

_____

_____

The first list is challenging, but the second may take even more effort. While you are keeping track of your feelings, I want you to also make an effort to track the times when what you are feeling differs from the face you are presenting to the world. For example, make notes of the times when you feel angry but put on a smiley face for the people around you or the times when you act indifferent to your sweetie but really want his or her warmth and attention. You'll be trying to catch yourself feeling one way and acting another. You'll be trying to notice yourself wearing masks, something we discuss in the next chapter. The purpose of this list is to help you see incongruities between how you feel and how you act and to bring more awareness to the masks you wear for the world.

_____

_____

_____

_____

_____

_____

_____

_____

You would think all the physical and emotional expenditures would be enough, but they are not. On top of all you are doing and feeling, you are probably worrying about things you are not doing or not feeling. That brings us to the next nonmonetary expenditure I want you to think about.

What, Me Worry?

From as far back as I can remember, my mother has been a master worrier. She worries about big things and little things, near things and far things, things she can control and things she can't. I even remember once hearing her worry aloud that she was worried about not having anything to worry about at the moment. For a time, she considered giving up amateur worrying to turn pro, but she worried about how she would look in the professional worrier's uniform and whether or not she would be good enough at fretting and fussing to get an endorsement deal.

During my first few years of life, many of her worries revolved around starting a family hundreds of miles away from her own parents—finances and the economy of the early 1970s being what they were—and the fact that my dad was in Vietnam trying not to get himself killed before his tour of duty was over. Her worrying rubbed off on me. I empathized with her, learned to worry from her during this time, and carried those worries with me to school. Remember, what we put out into the world comes back to us.

I was an anxious and insecure child, especially during those first few years of school. I worried about my big nose and pointy ears. I worried about what to say and what not to say. I worried about whether I walked right, talked right, and acted right around other kids and the teachers. All the worrying made me shy. I turned inward. I chewed up my shirt collars, gnawed on my fingernails, and licked and chomped my lips until they were raw and chapped.

I do not blame my mother for my awkwardness during those first years of school. I can indeed trace my propensity to worry back to her, but she is also the source of my desire to work with young children. Rather, it fascinates me that the stress and anxiety of the Vietnam era influenced my development. This might be a tad simplistic, but her worry over societal realities beyond her control and the lack of a healthy outlet for that worry wired itself into my busy brain.

The point is that worry can be as draining as our daily physical and emotional expenditures, and it can have a huge impact on our interactions with the children in our care. Again, what we put into the world comes back to us.

In my experience, worries seldom live up to the mental hype we give them. Our minds run wild and we blow small things out of proportion. My nose, though not small, is not something people bump into while walking down the street, and my ears, though a bit pointy, don't make strangers stop and point. So, in the end, we expend lots of time and energy giving our worries free and unfettered reign of our heads. I wish I could recapture all the time I worried about my nose and ears so I could devote it to things that are more useful. Spend some time thinking about your own worries:

What three things do you worry about most?

_____

_____

_____

What are the benefits of worrying about these things?

_____

_____

_____

What happens in your body when you are worried? What happens in your mind?

_____

_____

_____

What if you had no worries? How would you spend the time and energy you saved?

_____

_____

_____

What Do You Expect?

There was a need for a new vehicle at our house. I wanted a convertible. Tasha wanted a pickup. We got a pickup. We both noticed as we drove around town that we were seeing many pickups on the road, especially pickups that were the same color as ours, the same make and model as ours, or equipped with the same bed cover as ours. These trucks had always been there, but because our truck was front and center in our minds, we began seeing them. Our minds focused on the idea of *pickup* and were therefore primed to pick them out in traffic and parking lots.

We get what we expect from life. If your mind is primed to see pickups, you see pickups. If you expect to be miserable, miserable becomes easier to achieve. If you expect smiles, you get smiles. This is a simple concept, but powerful. Your mind holds on to the things you prime it to experience. With that in mind, take some time to answer the following questions:

What are you placing front and center in your mind and your life?

_____

_____

_____

Pay attention to your thoughts for a day. What are you saying to yourself about yourself? About other people or situations? Is it mostly positive, or mostly negative?

_____

_____

_____

Notice how your mind-set is impacting the people around you. How are they affected by your internal monologue?

_____

_____

_____

What Are Your Dreams?

In the time since I burned out at the job I loved and found family child care, I have also found an abundance of energy. I said earlier that I don't feel like what I do is work, but any rational look at my schedule would indicate I am accomplishing much more now than I was back at my old job. I have learned to take care of myself and, most importantly, take control of my stress. The biggest payoff is I now have the time, energy, and emotional balance to follow my dreams.

By identifying and then learning to manage the things that cause stress and zap energy, you free up resources to know and follow your dreams. Your dreams can give direction and focus to your life; they can give you purpose. They can also be energizing. Nothing motivates like a desire to achieve. Have you ever watched a two-year-old trying to get hold of a toy that is on a shelf a few inches higher than she can reach? The desire and drive glows in her eyes. Your eyes should have that same glow, and they will if you make an effort to know and follow your dreams. It is important that you spend some time thinking about what those dreams are as we move forward. For now, sit comfortably, close your eyes, and breathe deeply for a few moments. With your eyelids closed, start painting a picture of your life five years from now. Make the images as real as possible. Add sensory details: smells, sounds, feelings, tastes, sights, and feelings. Add motion. Make it as real as possible. When you are done, take a few moments to jot some notes about or draw a picture of your vision of the future in the space below.

Tactics, Tools, and Tips

1. Your physical exertions as a caregiver can leave you exhausted and lacking time for activities you enjoy. Making time for your favorite physical activities is a good tactic for maintaining your smile. Walking, gardening, running, yoga, karate, softball, and other vigorous pastimes get the blood flowing, energize the body, and release stress. Regularly investing a little time in physical exercise is a simple and sustainable way to improve your outlook.

2. Contemplate your job. What parts of it are the most stressful physically and emotionally? What parts of it bring you joy? If you could change it to be perfect for you, what would that look like? Don't worry about whether it's possible now, just imagine. Would you work part time? Have more authority? Have less responsibility? Just thinking about these things helps you better understand your situation and create a mind-set that is open to change. While you might be inclined to zoom off and make changes right away, I urge you to spend time thinking about your current situation. We sometimes rush into change and end up making things worse for ourselves by taking on too much too soon or by making the wrong changes for the right reasons.

3. Over the next few days, commit to an optimistic mind-set. When you catch yourself being negative or feeling down, make an effort to think positively. It is not easy if you are not used to it, so don't blame yourself if you have problems, and don't judge your success or failure. Just do your best at holding positive thoughts in your mind from moment to moment. Doing this is the beginning of retraining your mind and gaining control over your thinking.

   Here are some ways to change your outlook:

   • Look for the bright side of every situation. For example, if someone tracks mud on the floor, be happy it is not elephant dung. If someone cuts you off in traffic, be happy they did not hit you.

- When you notice you are telling someone off or going over an injustice in your mind, instead pay attention to something pleasurable—consciously turn your attention to the blue sky, beautiful trees, smile on a child's face, or something else that brings you contentment and peace.

- Take a moment to realize that, although you might be upset about something that happened in the past or that you fear in the future, in this moment you are safe and secure. Notice right now that you are okay.

Three

Knowing
Your Self

HOW WELL DO YOU *REALLY* know you? How well do you know your habits, understand your motivations, recognize the masks you wear, and identify with your "darkness"? How well do you know the *true* you?

I used to think I knew myself pretty well. Then, on a day that started out like any other day, I ended up quitting a job I had loved for sixteen years. My life kind of fell apart because I had become so consumed with my work that I lost track of who I really was. I had thought I knew what I wanted from life, what motivated me, what scared me, what my dreams were. I had thought I was tuned in to me, but I really wasn't. In truth, I was living a life of assumptions. A life barely examined below the surface. I thought I knew all about me, but I had never taken the time to examine my life thoughtfully, to really look below the surface—down deep—and back into the dark corners of myself.

Then again, why should I have? Life seemed to be going well, and looking below the surface of your life can be uncomfortable. Looking at your motivations, fears, ambitions, and dreams is not easy. That is why—if you are anything like me—you probably have not spent much time looking closely at yourself either. This chapter is devoted to taking a hard look at yourself.

Take a deep breath, and let's begin.

Do You Know Your Habits?

You are your habits. The way you talk, walk, solve problems, and address (or don't address) your stress are habits you have formed in your journey through life. Our habits are not good or bad; they just are. That being said, we all tend to classify habits into those two categories. Don't we? It's easy to blame our *bad* habits for our shortcomings, but our *good* habits can cause just as much trouble in our lives. In fact, our good habits can really make a mess of things. Sharing is a good habit. Right? Well, many caregivers share so much of their time, energy, and other resources that they have nothing left for themselves. Being selfless is a good habit too. Right? It's good to put the needs of others ahead of our own needs, but I know caregivers who have really mucked up their lives because they were too selfless.

You are your habits, and they can contribute to the stress, mental chatter, and outside pressure you experience as you skip, walk, or crawl through life. To put it bluntly, life sucks when your habits leave you feeling grouchy, gloomy, frazzled, or fried.

Forming habits takes time, and changing them requires thoughtful effort. I would like you to invest some time in contemplating your own habits:

What habits do you let control your life?

_____

_____

_____

When did each of the habits named above take hold?

_____

_____

_____

What one habit would you like to change the most? Why?

_____

_____

_____

What existing habits make you feel strong, capable, and powerful? Why?

_____

_____

_____

What new habit would make your life better? Why?

_____

_____

_____

What Is Your Purpose?

I have tried over the last few years to understand why professional caregivers choose to work with children, and I have discovered that caregivers can be divided into two main groups—the Ultimate Purpose group and the Unfulfilled group. Knowing which group you fit into is important because it helps you understand yourself a bit better and therefore leads you to make better choices as you work to maintain your smile.

THE ULTIMATE PURPOSE GROUP

When asked, most people I have met who intentionally entered the profession, who mostly enjoy their work, and who have been in the field for a long time claim they were "called to the work" or that it is their "reason for being." The reason so many people work in this profession for decades in spite of the well-documented low pay, poor benefits packages, lack of appreciation, limited opportunities for advancement, long hours, physical challenges, and emotional drain is that they feel it is their Ultimate Purpose. I hear stories about and explanations of this belief that include words such as passion, joy, delight, love, rewarding, respect, and smiles. I have also met many parents who describe parenting as their Ultimate Purpose and use very similar language to explain their belief. Some of us just feel we are meant to parent or work with children. I call this the Ultimate Purpose group.

Another thing I have noticed about the Ultimate Purpose group is I can divide them into two subgroups. Some feel called to caregiving because they want to recreate the thrill of their own childhood, and others feel called to repair past wrongs. Some want to remake magical childhoods for the children in their life; others want to prevent in the lives of the kids they care for the pain, hurt, abuse, and sorrow they've experienced. I was a nervous, twitchy kid for part of my childhood, but overall it was a great time full of love, play, exploration, and fun. Tasha and I have worked hard to recreate those great times for the two children we have made and for all the kids we have cared for in the last twenty plus years. Others have had different experiences. I have heard chilling stories of physical and sexual abuse, abandonment, and parental apathy that have led people to devote their lives to caring for young children. This is in no way scientific, but perhaps if you allow yourself a moment, you will quickly decide which group is yours. Knowing which of these groups you fit into may not seem important at first. In fact, it may mean thinking about things you would rather not think about and dealing with feelings you would rather ignore. Knowing which group you fit into provides some insight into your professional choices and your personal actions and reactions. Understanding why we do what we do can also be very empowering. No matter why we believe it, some of us feel called to work with children; we feel it is our Ultimate Purpose.

In my experience, I've found it is easy for this group of people to get lost in their calling. They give themselves so fully that their work as caregiver or parent completely consumes their personal identity. They do not take care of their own needs because they are so busy taking care of the people around them. Their work swallows them whole.

Close your eyes and take a few long breaths. Now look deep inside yourself and think about if you are a member of the Ultimate Purpose group. Do you feel your work as a caregiver or parent is your calling in life? If so, consider the following questions:

What steps are you taking to keep your head clear and your mind focused on that calling?

_____

_____

_____

_____

Why do you think caregiving is your Ultimate Purpose?

_____

_____

_____

_____

THE UNFULFILLED GROUP

If you do not feel called to be a caregiver, working with children long term is probably more challenging. It is hard to do something year after year when you are not passionate about it. It's challenging to do work that does not feed your soul in some way. I have met many caregivers who have worked in the field for decades despite loathing their jobs. I have also met parents who did not want children and do not like parenting. I am not judging these people. In fact, I have met many parents and caregivers who would put themselves in this category who are very good at nurturing, teaching, and caring. As a group, they just do not find the work as fulfilling, meaningful, and important as those who feel their work is also their purpose. Some feel they have abandoned their personal dreams and goals. Some feel they blinked and a huge chunk of life zipped past. Some are just lost souls drifting through their own existence. I call this the Unfulfilled group.

Members of the Ultimate Purpose group can lose themselves in their work, and members of the Unfulfilled group often just feel lost. Those in the Unfulfilled group do not know what their Ultimate Purpose is, or they know what it is but believe it is unattainable. They may have lost their love for children and child care after unappreciated and underpaid years of work. The realities of parenting may not be what they expected. They may feel stuck in a job they took because it was the only thing available. If you are a member of this group, you may need to make major changes to maintain your smile. You may need to change your career. You deserve to live your Ultimate Purpose too. You just might have to work to figure out what it is and how to live it.

If you didn't classify yourself as a member of the Ultimate Purpose group, you are a member of the Unfulfilled group by default. That's okay. It's not bad to be in this group. It just means that much of the stress you currently have or that could develop comes from a different place. Spending a huge part of your life doing something that is not your passion is a great way to add stress to your life and fade your smile. If you are a member of this group, what you need most is to know what your Ultimate Purpose is, and then make changes so you can live that purpose. Consider the following questions:

When you close your eyes and envision your perfect life, what are you doing? If caregiving is not your Ultimate Purpose, what is?

_____

_____

_____

How did you end up as a caregiver? Was it something you pursued or was it an accident?

_____

_____

_____

What career would bring you the most joy, happiness, and smiles?

_____

_____

_____

CLOAK OF TRANQUILITY

When you picture the Cloak of Tranquility, picture Harry Potter's Cloak of Invisibility with a few added features. Not only does the Cloak of Tranquility make you invisible, it snuggles up against you and helps you calm down. It relaxes you with a variety of techniques, including aromatherapy, three types of massage, acupuncture, guided imagery, and white noise. Not only do you become invisible to the world, you are also wrapped in a cozy cocoon of relaxation programmed to calm and soothe your tattered nerves.

The _Deluxe_ Cloak of Tranquility comes with a tranquility timer that buzzes after a preselected time period to remind you that there is an outside world that needs you. It also has a reading light so you can catch up on your reading and a minirefrigerator/freezer for snacks. The Cloak of Tranquility is now available in a variety of fabrics. Dry clean only.

Do You Know Your Masks?

We all wear masks for the world. On any given day, I might put on my Husband mask, Father mask, Son mask, Child Care Professional mask, Leave Me Alone mask, Author mask, Speaker mask, Yoga Instructor mask, Outraged Citizen mask, Concerned Citizen mask, and Jerk mask. The masks we wear represent different aspects of our personalities and different personas we want the world to see. We use them to protect ourselves, to market ourselves, and to empower ourselves. Our masks can assist and hinder. They can harm and help. They can push people away, and they can pull people near. In and of themselves, masks are neither good nor bad. They just are. But sometimes we use them in unhealthy, harmful, or hurtful ways.

Sometimes there are huge differences among our masks, and sometimes they cause conflict in our heads and lives. When I was in college, I worked the overnight shift at a convenience store on weekends. It was a very interesting job that gave me an opportunity to meet many kinds of people. In particular, I looked forward to seeing the strippers—two or three beautiful young women who danced at the Pink Pussy Cat down the street. They came in every night after their shift for convenience store food, including microwave burritos, stale nachos, or over-cooked hotdogs. They were tired, colorful, talkative, sarcastic, and fun. They would hang out for twenty or thirty minutes—eating and chatting about their night. One dancer frequently offered to flash me as payment for her $1.29 nachos, claiming it was a slow night and she did not have any dollar bills.

One night there was a new dancer with the regulars who was one of my classmates from college. She was as shocked to see me as I was to see her. There was immediate conflict between her stripper mask and her college student mask. Her eyeballs popped out of her head (just like in the cartoons) when she saw me. While the other women were foraging for grub, she begged me in a whisper, *"Please,* don't tell anyone." I assured her that her secret was safe. But, eventually, her secret did get out; someone less discreet from school started talking. At that point, she could no longer separate the two masks or the lives that went with them.

The more conflict there is between our masks, the more trouble we have reconciling the lives they represent. Before I burned out and learned to live a more mindful life, there were huge differences between my various masks. I often had to stop and think about which persona I needed to present to which people. Since I have made an effort to take better physical and emotional care of myself, I have noticed that my masks are not as different from one another as they once were. I am more balanced.

Our masks can be hindrances: they can keep us from dealing with issues we need to address, they can help us hide from issues that need attention, and they can block open and honest communication. Becoming aware of your masks can help you recognize when your masks are holding you back. Most of us are more likely to use masks to hide from reality than we are to use them to change our reality. It is easy to hide behind your collection of masks until you lose yourself. It is easy to wear a particular set of defensive masks so long that you forget you are wearing them. Over time, the happy-face mask you wear for the world begins to chafe. Conflict arises between the face you put on for the world and the way you really feel down deep. We all know people who are happy campers for the world while they are falling apart inside.

If you use them consciously, masks can help you out. For example, I currently spend over half my weekends away from home speaking at conferences and training events around the U.S. and abroad. I enjoy it, and I am good at it. That has not always been the case. Remember high school and how you had to get up and do a sixty-second speech in front of the class? Well, I was so nervous that I chose a lower grade in the class over getting up and talking. I was simply too scared—too paralyzed—to do it. It's not uncommon; lots of people are frightened to speak in front of groups.

To overcome my fear, I made myself a confident speaker mask, put it on, and started volunteering to give presentations. I did everything I could to present a strong, in-control face to the world while I was nearly vomiting in my mouth every time I stood in front of a group. I remember feeling lightheaded, sick, and weak the first time I spoke to a group of child care providers at a conference. It was a struggle to make it through the sixty-minute presentation. Over time, the mask helped me gain the confidence I needed. It helped me change the habit of fear, and it helped me move toward my dreams and goals. Masks can be used to make you stronger and to transform your life.

I want you to spend some time thinking about your masks so that you have more choices for using them. Here are some activities and questions to help increase awareness of your masks. Think about them, and then write your responses on the lines that follow:

- Make a list of all the masks you wear for the world.
- Next to each mask list the people you wear it for.

- Next to each mask estimate how much time each week you spend wearing it.

- On a scale of one to ten, rate each mask on how close it is to the "real" you. One equals "almost the real me" and ten equals "I'm really acting when I wear this one."

- Spend some time thinking about why you wear each of your masks. Which of them could you do without? Which needs refitting? What new masks might you want to add to your collection?

_____

_____

_____

_____

_____

Are You Acknowledging Your Darkness?

Our tendency is to suppress and ignore our fear, pain, hurt, turmoil, angst, stress, rage, depression, anger, melancholy, regret, discomfort, worry, embarrassment, sadness, and grief. Most of us do our best to ignore our inner darkness. Instead of experiencing these things and then letting them go, we stuff them deep down inside and try to ignore them. Publicly feeling these things is generally taboo, and most of us don't have experience expressing them in healthy ways. We opt for suppression. We feel uncomfortable sharing them with the people closest to us, so there is no way we will let them out in public. We hide our darkness, believing it will go away if ignored long enough, and strap on a happy face for the world.

We carry around little things that irritate us and big things that have hurt us badly. Some of what we carry has happened recently, and other things have been weighing on us for years, even decades. I have swallowed anger over being cut off in traffic and let it eat at me for hours, and I have carried grudges against friends and foes, for real and imagined wrongs, for decades. You build walls, wear masks, and exert lots of energy trying to pretend it is not there. You may think ignoring your darkness has made it disappear, only to become enraged or burst into tears when life randomly trips an emotional trigger. Your darkness is powerful, and you can become lost in its inky depths if you are not careful.

Getting to know your darkness takes away its power. Acknowledging that it exists is a step toward weakening its control over you. The previous sentence was going to start "Simply acknowledging that it exists" or "Just acknowledging that it exists," but that made such an acknowledgment sound easier than it often is. Connecting with the smaller bits and pieces of your darkness may be simple, but it takes some work to open up to the bigger things you may be carrying. When you know your darkness, you not only take away its power, you also begin to feel lighter and more present in your life. It is easier to move through the present without the weight of the past hindering your every step.

We look at dealing with your darkness later; now, I just want you to get to know it a bit better. Use the space provided to make a list of your darkness—the life experiences and feelings that you ignore, suppress, and hide from:

- List every darkness you can think of, large and small. You may not be able to make a complete list all at once. That's okay. Add to the list as things come to mind. Consider spending a few minutes just sitting and breathing deeply to clear your head and see what things pop into your mind.

- As you build your list, estimate how long you have been carrying each item with you and make a note about this.

- Also make notes about why the items on your list still weigh on you and how they affect your interactions with people who are important to you.

_____

_____

_____

_____

What Are You Doing Right?

This chapter has asked some pretty heavy questions and, at this point, you may feel a bit overwhelmed by some of the things I have asked you to think about in an effort to know yourself better. While thinking about these things is important, knowing yourself better also means taking a close look at all the things (and I am sure there are a lot of them) that you are doing right. Knowing your successful choices, your healthy practices, and your positive activities is just as important as knowing your masks and your darkness. One thing that happens to a lot of people when they first begin to get overcome by their stress and burnout is that they abandon (or ignore) the successful, healthy, positive parts of their life. They may stop exercising, begin paying less attention to what they eat, pull away from friends and family, or abandon activities that recharged them at the end of tough days.

Keeping the successes in your life front and center in your mind helps you appreciate them—and it makes it harder for them to slip away when life gets stressful. Here are some activities that help you know more about your successes. Once you've completed them, you can reference your answers when life gets tough and you need a reminder of the good things in your life:

List your five proudest moments in the last six months.

_____

_____

_____

_____

_____

List ten nonwork activities, functions, or hobbies that bring you the most joy during your week.

_____

_____

_____

_____

_____

_____

_____

Which of your accomplishments from last year are you are most proud of?

_____

_____

_____

_____

_____

What are your biggest successes?

_____

_____

_____

_____

_____

Describe your most successful and healthy relationships.

_____

_____

_____

_____

_____

Do You Notice Your Joy?

Before wrapping up this chapter, the final thing I want you to consider is your *joy*. Even when life is flowing along smoothly, most of us fail to spend much time contemplating the things in life that bring us joy. When life gets challenging—when you step on a Cheerio in your bare feet, when you worry that the car payment you mailed on Monday might make it to the bank before the deposit you made on Wednesday, when you notice a bruise on a child that doesn't look accidental—your joy starts to slip from your mind. The worse your stress gets and the more submerged in it you become, the less likely you are to notice the activities, people, and things that bring happiness and joy into your life.

One of my biggest regrets in life is that I missed so much of the joy that emanated from my wife and children while I was burning out. It was there, but I just failed to see much of it. You can't get those moments back. That is why it is important for you to know what brings you joy, and then to hold on to it tightly—especially when life gets tough. The following questions and activities are to help you know your joy so that you can hold on to it when you need it most:

What three things about your work bring you the most joy?

_____

_____

_____

_____

What three activities away from work bring the most joy to your life?

_____

_____

_____

_____

Who are the people in your life that you spend most of your joyful moments with? Why do you believe these people are tied so closely to your joy?

_____

_____

_____

_____

Spend a few moments with your eyes closed, visualizing a joyful moment from the last month. Then use the space provided to describe your feelings and physical sensations associated with that moment.

_____

_____

_____

_____

Go through your photo albums, hard drive, or that shoe box in your closet and find a few pictures of faces that bring joy to your life. Then hang those pictures in a location where you will see them when you need a reminder of your joy.

Tactics, Tools, and Tips

1. Review your answers to the questions in the first three chapters, or go back and complete them if you zipped past them while reading. Think about what those answers mean to you. How do they relate to the realities of your daily life? My hope is that you have opened your mind a bit to the things that are stealing your smile and sucking up your physical and emotional energy. Being aware of these things is a necessary first step in dealing with them. Now take a small second step. Choose one small change you can make in your life right now that will lessen your stress or bring a smidgen more joy into your day.

2. Make an effort to be more aware, or more mindful, of how you move through the world and interact with the people and things around you. Habits are hard to change, but they're impossible to change if you are unaware of them. Try this:

- Clasp your hands by weaving your fingers together and bringing your palms together, like people do when they are praying.

- Look at your pinkies. Is your left pinky on the bottom or is your right pinky?

- Unclasp your hands and clasp them together again, shifting all your fingers so that your other pinky is on the bottom.

3. How does it feel to have your fingers folded differently? People have described it to me as wrong, odd, awkward, different, uncomfortable, unnatural, and painful. I've even met a few people who could not physically do this activity because their habitual way of doing it was so ingrained in their minds that their fingers would not cooperate when they tried to do it the "wrong" way. One woman had to have a friend help her arrange her fingers. I want you to know that all the words used to describe the feeling of rearranged fingers also describe what you feel when you make other, bigger changes. Change is not easy; the first step is mindfulness.

With that in mind, start practicing being aware of your thoughts and feelings.

4. Go do something you enjoy. Be a bit selfish. I know you don't think you have time for yourself. I know you don't think it is right to put yourself ahead of the children in your life. I know you think doing things just for yourself is selfish. Get over it! That thinking weakens your smile.

Four

Picking
Your Purpose

SO FAR A LOT OF PAGES have been devoted to the whys and hows of stress and burnout. Those readers who are currently experiencing these things have probably recognized signs and symptoms of their own burnout. Readers who are not currently burned out have gotten a glimpse of where they are headed if they don't take action and begin caring for themselves more thoughtfully. I know caregivers who have spent years struggling in a frantic state of stress until they broke down and left the profession. Some knew they were stressed but were unable—or unwilling—to do anything about it. Others did not even see their stress until it had taken over and driven them from the profession.

I have also known caregivers who thought they were invulnerable to any kind of stress or burnout. One woman I met a few years ago insisted that she thrived on the stress that came from pushing herself so hard. She worked full time in a center-based program, taught Sunday school, coached a soccer team, volunteered at her children's school, and did lots of other job-related volunteer work. Six months after the conference at which she had gone on and on about how she was stressed but in total control and thriving on that stress, I received an e-mail from her informing me that she had quit her job and left her husband because she "couldn't take it any longer."

No matter how super-human you may feel, you are indeed vulnerable to the stress in your life. Understanding where that stress comes from and how it can influence your life is the first step. Now I want to begin looking at what you can do to take control of your life.

Are You Making the Most of Your Dash?

I plan to die smiling on July 15, 2094, while celebrating the 108th anniversary of the first time Tasha kissed me. It happens at sunset during a romantic encounter in an orange and purple striped hot air balloon high above Easter Island in the South Pacific. Below, silent rows of giant Maori keep their eyes to themselves, stoically staring out to sea. A pod of whales slips silently by, consumed with the pursuit of plankton in the calm, glassy sea. We die in each other's arms after ninety-two years, six months, and thirteen days of marriage with a kiss as sweet and gentle as the first one, drifting along as the balloon slowly loses altitude. I will be 125 years old.

A vacationing family from Seattle finds our bodies and the tattered balloon a few weeks later while looking at kangaroos in southwestern Australia. The parents each say a few kind words over our bodies before strapping us to the top of their rented Range Rover and hauling us back to Sydney. Their two children hardly lift their eyes from their holographic video games. Once in Sydney, the family contacts our children and asks what to do with us. Tyler and Zoë instruct them to have us cremated and shipped home.

The crematorium has some problems. Our bodies are so dried out and stiff after two weeks in the blazing sun that they are unable to disentwine us. We look like two twisted hunks of beef jerky. They give up trying to separate us and cremate us together. Then we are packaged and shipped home in a single urn engraved as shown here:

Jeff A. Johnson
&
Tasha A. Johnson
1969–2094

They Died Smiling

Read the engraving on that urn again and look at those dates. That seemingly inconsequential dash between the years 1969 and 2094 engraved on that urn represents our lives. It represents every moment between our first and last breaths, every choice, every action, every inaction, every hesitation, every leap of faith, every intention, every dream deferred or fulfilled, every kiss, every step, every second of life. In the end, all the joy and heartache, accomplishments and failures, easy and hard times, smiles and tears, mountains and mole hills, smooth sailing and stressful struggles we experience during our lives gets whittled down to a dash.

We tend to take life completely for granted, wrongfully assuming we have all the time in the world. We drift aimlessly like that orange and purple striped hot air balloon until torn to tatters by the realization that life is limited. We get bogged down in the day to day of our lives and fail to think about who we really are and what we are doing. I spent the first thirty-four years of my life mostly drifting. I had some direction and drive, but mostly I let life happen to me. I spent more time reacting to life than living it purposefully.

Since burning out, I have found my purpose. I have learned to make the most of my dash. Chances are you are so caught up in meeting the needs of others that you don't even think about what *you* need. This chapter is about naming what *you* need from *your* life. It is about finding the reason for *your* dash. It is about finding *your* Ultimate Purpose. Life is short. What are you going to do with your dash?

What's Your Purpose?

Eight activities intended to get you thinking about your Ultimate Purpose follow. You can do them all, or you can choose to do the ones that appeal to you most. What is important is that you devote time to trying to define your purpose. If you already know your purpose revolves around working with children, use these activities to help refine your thinking. If you think your Ultimate Purpose lies elsewhere, use these tools to help figure out how you should really be spending your dash.

As you do these activities, I implore you to be honest with yourself. Editing your thoughts, feelings, ideas, and dreams to fit someone else's mold is not going to help you identify *your* purpose. Your Ultimate Purpose in life is not determined by what your parents, sweetheart, child, friends, or neighbors think; it is something you have to find for yourself inside your own head. Be a bit selfish here, take off all your masks, and try to gain a deeper understanding of your true self. You deserve to spend some time candidly contemplating your own existence.

Why is identifying your Ultimate Purpose so important? It makes you powerful and gives you more control in your day-to-day life. It defines you, it clarifies your thinking, and it gives you direction. Think of your Ultimate Purpose as a lighthouse off in the distance that you can always see when you feel adrift in the world. It shows you which direction to go. When faced with a difficult decision, your purpose guides you toward the choice that is most in line with your truest self. Whenever I feel challenged or beat up by life, I visualize my Ultimate Purpose. It gives me the strength to muscle through tough situations, the calm to think clearly, and the focus to make good choices.

Take a couple of those deep, cleansing breaths, and get to know yourself better.

NAMING YOUR PURPOSE

On the lines that follow, answer this question: What is my Ultimate Purpose? Write any answer that snaps, crackles, or pops into your head. Your answer may be a detailed paragraph or it may be a single word or phrase. The size of your answer doesn't matter—getting it on the page is what is important. Now keep writing down answers to the question "What is my Ultimate Purpose?" until you respond emotionally to one of your answers. It may bring tears, it may bring a sigh of relief, it may bring a sense of calm, it may just feel right. You know you are close to naming your Ultimate Purpose when you experience a strong emotional connection to your answer.

_____

_____

_____

_____

_____

_____

_____

_____

_____

_____

_____

MEETING BUD

Suppose that one morning while you are preparing to brush your teeth a genie appears from your toothpaste tube and announces, "My name is Bud the Genie, and I am here to grant you one wish." What would you wish for? Take some time to think, come up with a good answer and write it down:

_____

_____

_____

_____

_____

As you are finishing making your wish, you realize that Bud limited you to only one wish, but he did not put any limits on that wish. Since genies don't regularly pop out of your toothpaste, you decide to make the most of this unique situation and see how much you can get from him. You decide to add an *and* to the end of your wish instead of a period so that you can just keep on wishing. Bud does not seem to object, so you keep on wishing:

AND I want . . .

AND I want . . .

_____

AND I want . . .

_____

AND for my sweetie I want . . .

_____

AND for my family I want . . .

_____

AND for the people next door I want . . .

_____

AND for my community I want . . .

_____

AND for the clerk at the gas station I want . . .

_____

AND for the hermit cat lady down the street I want . . .

_____

AND for that guy I don't know that just drove by I want . . .

_____

AND for _____ I want . . .

_____

AND for _____ I want . . .

_____

You know what you want from Bud and have an idea what people close to you may want, but as you start making wishes for the gas station clerk, the cat lady, and the stranger driving by it becomes impossible to know what they want. Your wishes for those people have more to do with what you have to give than what they want—and what you have to give has a great deal to do with your Ultimate Purpose. Over the next few days, imagine what you would wish for the strangers you see. Look for themes and connections in your wishes for them. Think about how these wishes for strangers relate to your Ultimate Purpose.

LOOKING AT YOUR PAST

In this exercise, I want you to take some time to look back at different periods in your life and try to determine if there are some common themes and interests. Please use the space provided to answer the following questions for each period of your life:

CHILDHOOD

What were your favorite activities?

_____

_____

_____

Were you a leader or a follower?

_____

What things most interested you?

_____

_____

_____

Where was your favorite place during this time of your life?

_____

_____

What kinds of people did you prefer?

_____

_____

How physically active were you?

_____

_____

When were you happiest?

_____

_____

When were you most sad?

_____

_____

ADOLESCENCE

What were your favorite activities?

_____

_____

_____

Were you a leader or a follower?

_____

What things most interested you?

_____

_____

_____

Where was your favorite place during this time of your life?

_____

_____

What kinds of people did you prefer?

_____

_____

How physically active were you?

_____

_____

When were you happiest?

_____

_____

When were you most sad?

_____

_____

ADULTHOOD

What are your favorite activities?

_____

_____

_____

Are you a leader or a follower?

_____

What things most interest you?

_____

_____

_____

Where is your favorite place?

_____

_____

What kinds of people do you prefer?

_____

_____

How physically active are you?

_____

_____

When are you happiest?

_____

_____

When are you most sad?

_____

_____

Review your answers, looking for commonalities and themes, and then spend some time connecting them to your current life. Then look at how you live life day to day. You may see some life-long interests that you have overlooked or suppressed. You may realize you have drifted away from things you enjoy. You may recognize that you have always been a physically active person and are unhappy being tied to an overly sedentary job. You may realize you prefer to be alone and have a career that requires you to be a "people person," or you may just admit to yourself that your daily life does not include many of the things that have always made you happy. Use your answers to the questions in this activity to help refine your Ultimate Purpose.

DREAMING YOUR DREAMS

This activity allows you to better understand your Ultimate Purpose by looking at your dreams for the future. Spend a few moments breathing deeply and then answer each of these questions. Don't spend a lot of time thinking about the question, just jot down the first answer that pops into your mind:

What kinds of people do you want to surround yourself with?

_____

_____

_____

What places do you want to visit?

_____

_____

What career changes will you make in the next five years?

_____

_____

_____

What hobbies do you plan to pursue?

_____

_____

What do you want to learn more about?

_____

_____

_____

How do you plan to use the wisdom you have accumulated in life?

_____

_____

_____

Who will you be spending most of your time with five years from now?

_____

_____

_____

Review your answers to the questions. In the space provided, note any emerging themes or connections that may relate to your Ultimate Purpose.

_____

_____

_____

_____

_____

IDENTIFYING WHAT YOU CAN'T STAND

Knowing what you don't like in your current situation can help bring what you really want into focus. For example, if you are regularly upset about your long commute to and from your job, then finding work closer to home (or a home closer to work) may relieve a huge amount of stress. In this exercise, you are going to look at what you don't like and try to figure out what you want instead.

You are going to divide your life into two categories—work life and home life. Your job is to use the space provided to list what you can't stand about each area of your life and then describe what you would prefer it to be like. When listing the things you can't stand, please be honest with yourself. Let it out. Admit what you feel. You can safely remove your content employee and happy homemaker masks for this activity. When you describe how you would prefer things to be, dream big! The only way to make real progress is to be fully honest with yourself.

WORK LIFE

I can't stand . . .

_____

_____

I would prefer . . .

_____

_____

HOME LIFE

I can't stand . . .

_____

_____

I would prefer . . .

_____

_____

IMAGINING WHAT OTHERS WOULD SAY

Imagine celebrating your 110th birthday surrounded by friends, admirers, and loved ones. You have lived a long, productive, healthy, and happy life. Before blowing out all the candles on an elaborate cake, a number of speakers get up to make short speeches about you. Visualize each of the following people and what they have to say. Use the space provided to write down their words:

Your sweetie . . .

_____

_____

_____

Your child . . .

_____

_____

_____

A long-time coworker . . .

_____

_____

_____

The mayor of your community . . .

_____

_____

_____

Your best friend . . .

_____

_____

_____

As you review what you have written, consider how it relates to your Ultimate Purpose in life. Are you on track to make their words reality, or do you need to make changes in your life? If change is needed, what do you need to change?

HANGING WITH BUD AGAIN

Suppose that Bud the Genie appears again the next time you brush your teeth with Aladdin's Tooth Gel ("1,000 magic smiles in every tube") and offers to make your life perfect. All he asks is that you provide a detailed description of what your perfect life would look like. Use the space provided to explain your perfect life. Consider the following in your answer:

- What are your surroundings like?
- How do you spend your time?
- What do you have more of and less of?
- What do you give up?
- How do you interact with the world?
- What do you enjoy and love?
- How do you feel?

_____

_____

_____

_____

_____

_____

MAKING YOUR LIST

I stated the obvious at the beginning of the chapter when I said life is short. It is something we all know all too well, yet most of us spend absurd amounts of time watching television, worrying, and waiting for life to happen to us. We find it very difficult to take control of our lives and live like every moment matters.

In this exercise, I want you to list everything you want to accomplish, experience, and achieve before reaching the end of your dash. Do you want to skinny-dip with your sweetie at sunset in the Caribbean? Put it on the list. Do you want to learn to juggle? Add it to your list. Do you want to earn a PhD? List it. Do you want to learn to weld? Write it down! Use the space provided to list the things you want to do before you die. Fold the corner of the page to mark it, then look back frequently to check things off your list or add new ideas.

_____

_____

_____

_____

_____

QUESTIONING YOURSELF

Here are a few final questions to contemplate. Take your time with them:

What price are you paying for not pursuing your Ultimate Purpose?

_____

_____

_____

What changes are you willing to make in order to live your Ultimate Purpose?

_____

_____

_____

What cause are you willing to dedicate your life to?

_____

_____

_____

What activities do you engage in or discuss with others, during which you lose all track of time?

_____

_____

_____

What Is My Purpose?

Next I'm going to ask you to write down your Ultimate Purpose based on what you have learned about yourself in the preceding activities. Before you get to that, I think it is important that I provide some tips to help you write it effectively.

Keep It Short

The mission statement of Google, a huge international company, is only fifteen words long: Google's mission is "to organize the world's information and make it universally accessible and useful." If Google can state their Ultimate Purpose in a short sentence, you should be able to do the same. Keeping it short is challenging. It means you have to work to clarify and refine your thinking. Keeping it short also makes it easier to remember.

Make It Visual

To me, Google gets this right too. I can see a picture in my head of a world where all information is universally accessible and useful. When you write your Ultimate Purpose, try to use language that creates a strong mental image.

Say It Clearly

Leave out technical or professional jargon. Use simple, concrete words. Google's mission statement does not say a thing about server farms, Boolean logic, or packet jams. Your statement of Ultimate Purpose shouldn't be filled with jargon. Yours is a loftier pursuit.

Make It Honest

Your Ultimate Purpose is meaningless unless you are completely honest with yourself while writing it. If it is to have any meaning in your life, it has to be _YOUR_ purpose.

Your Ultimate Purpose should not be set in stone. It needs to flex and evolve over time as your life changes. Every year or two you should invest some time in reviewing your statement of purpose and see if it is still accurate. Leave it alone if it is still truthful, and revise it if needed. This statement is your guiding light. It is important for it to always be fresh and meaningful.

Using the tips given, write your statement of Ultimate Purpose:

_____

_____

_____

_____

_____

_____

_____

_____

What Are Your Goals?

Now that you know your purpose in life, it is important you take steps to live that purpose. This means setting some SMART goals. SMART goals are goals that are

Specific (Who, what, where, when, why, and/or how?)

Measurable (How will you measure success?)

Attainable (Can you really achieve this goal?)

Results-oriented (Does this goal bring you closer to living your Ultimate Purpose?)

Time-bound (What's the deadline?)

For example, if living your Ultimate Purpose requires that you go back to school, two possible goals may be (1) By June 1, I will investigate enrollment options at all local colleges, and (2)

By the end of July, I will complete and submit a college application. Both of these goals include information about who does what and when. They are measurable, they are doable, they fit the purpose, and they are time-bound. Please note that if you write a goal that does not seem attainable, you may just be taking too big a bite. Consider breaking such goals down into smaller, bite-size pieces.

Use the space provided to write three to five short-term goals that get you a few steps closer to living your Ultimate Purpose.

_____

_____

_____

_____

_____

_____

Tactics, Tools, and Tips

1. A little self-care on a regular basis is far better than a lot of self-care every once in a while. It is easy to forget about a once-a-week commitment, or allow life to bulldoze it out of your schedule. Do you brush your teeth and hair once a week for a long time or do you brush them for a short amount of time every day? Doing a little of something every day helps it become a habit. Devoting five or ten minutes every day to meeting your own needs benefits you more than spending an hour on it once a week. Make a daily self-care habit like caring for your teeth and hair. Your emotional well-being deserves at least as much of your focused, daily attention as your teeth and hair, doesn't it? What you do is up to you, but it should be something that helps you focus, charges you up for the day, or just makes you feel good. I do yoga and meditate every morning, but I know people who do things such as run, read, listen to music, garden, pray, and sew. What is important is that you find something you enjoy and can commit to.

2. Is this worthwhile? Is this the best use of my dash? Is this part of my Ultimate Purpose? Make it a habit to ask yourself these questions before taking on new projects, obligations, and responsibilities. If you answer *no* to these questions, you may want to consider saying no to the project, obligation, or responsibility.

3. Now that you have clearly stated your Ultimate Purpose, you need to remember that you can create new masks to help you live that purpose. Living your purpose may mean building new habits or taking on new roles. These things can be easier if you spend some time thinking about what kinds of masks you need to achieve your goals. For example, in the section on goals, I used going back to college as an example of something you may do in pursuit of your Ultimate Purpose. That scenario also may require some special masks, especially if you have been away from a formal learning environment for a while. You may need a confident student mask or a dedicated learner mask. The point is if you need a mask to move forward in life take the time to make it, and then use it as needed. It could really help mend your mind-set, and that's what chapter five is all about.

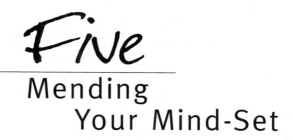

Five
Mending
Your Mind-Set

MY FRIEND CHRIS BLADES HELPED me mend my mind-set. You may
have read about him in my book *Finding Your Smile Again.* He was
an elementary school custodian by day and a tae kwon do instructor in the evenings. He was probably the best and most natural
teacher I have ever met, because he was able to tune in to his
students as individuals. What my daughter Zoë learned from him
in class has helped make her strong, confident, kind, and determined. He knew I was burning out at my center job before I knew
and told me to let go and enjoy life. He introduced me to yoga and
meditation and inspired me to live my Ultimate Purpose.

Chris helped me realize I could make changes in my life.
He taught me that I could overcome obstacles and live the life I
wanted if I acted thoughtfully, let go of the things I allowed to
hold me back, and trusted my intuition. He helped me get comfortable in my own head by showing me how to let go of the
constant clutter and chatter that was going on in there. His unaf-
fected, laid-back manner and his forthrightness coupled with his
joy for life made him easy to talk to and listen to. He also lived
his words. He was far from perfect, but he was constantly working to be a better person: tweaking his diet, trying to improve
his attitude, attempting to live a more complete life.

You may have noticed I am talking about him in the past
tense.

The morning of April 18, 2007, a few days before *Finding Your Smile Again*'s release, I received a phone call from a friend informing me that Chris had died the night before. I did not believe her. For a few minutes, I was sure it was a well-planned and intentionally late April Fools' Day joke meant to catch me off guard. Chris was in great physical shape. He lifted weights, did lots of cardio, ate well, meditated every day, dealt well with his stress, got enough sleep, and didn't smoke. He lived the way experts say to live if you want a long, healthy life. It took my friend about five minutes to make me believe he was really gone.

He had an undiagnosed hereditary heart condition. He had been lying in bed with his hand on his dog's head watching *The Andy Griffith Show* on TV Land when his heart failed, and he died. His wife came home from work. She started talking to him, but he did not reply. She walked into the bedroom and found him, his hand still resting on the dog's head. He was fifty-one.

I'm not the only one Chris inspired. His visitation and memorial service were standing room only. The building was overflowing with people wanting to honor their memories of the life he lived. I have never seen as many tough, manly men brought to tears as I did at those two events honoring Chris's life. If that little dash between our date of birth and date of death represents our life then Chris Blades lived one hell of a dash.

I really don't know if he intended to teach me all the things I learned from him, but I learned them from him anyway. I do know he lived a life devoted to his wife, daughter, family, friends, and God. His life was full of martial arts, bow hunting, cycling, camping, yoga, and meditation. I don't think he set out to influence, encourage, inspire, motivate, and empower so many people, but he did. He was just living his life, and it was an inspiring life that touched lots of people. It was not a big, fancy, public life; it was not a life of fame or fortune. I think he was mostly just a guy, trying to live the best life he could, who happened to radiate a positive, hopeful, joyful energy that people readily responded to.

My mind-set changed as I learned to emulate his positive, hopeful, and joyful outlook. I gave up a pessimistic, sarcastic, cynical, and angry mind-set in favor of one that is freer, less judgmental, and more positive. I abandoned some unhealthy masks and cobbled together a few that are more in line with my new outlook. I quit trying to control everything, and I've become more open to life. I dumped my distrust and suspicion. I decided that my life works better if I trust people and the universe as a whole.

These changes in my mind-set did not happen overnight. I am a work in progress. I have worked for years to discard old habits and develop new ones. I used to think I was a finished product, incapable of change. Over the last few years, I have become more flexible and open to different ideas and new opportunities. Giving up rigidity for flexibility and reticence for openness has taken time. It hasn't been easy either. I've had to abandon pieces of myself that had become outdated and replace them with pieces that better fit my new mind-set. For example, I used to use mean-spirited sarcasm to belittle and marginalize people who held views different from mine. I did this to protect my beliefs and shelter my fragile ego. It was a very effective tool, but as I have grown more open to other people's ideas and beliefs, it has become less necessary. Now when confronted with a new idea or opinion, I opt to listen carefully and evaluate it based on merit instead of closing my mind and dismissively reaching for sarcasm . . . well . . . most of the time. Sometimes I still find myself shutting down and muttering something sarcastic under my breath. Like I said, I am a work in progress, and changing my mind-set is not easy. The best I can do is consciously strive to evolve into the person I want to become.

Before Chris taught me to open my mind to new opportunities, stop judging others (and myself) so harshly, enjoy life as it comes, and realize I did not always have to be in control, I was on a road to burnout that would have led me away from a profession I love. Changing my mind-set renewed my passion for early care and education and refocused my life. Adjusting your mind-set can do the same for you. Being conscious of what is going on inside your head helps you maintain your direction if you know where you are going, and it helps you find your direction if you are drifting.

Can You Find Your Inner Judge?

Altering your mind-set requires regular attention to your actions. Changing the way you see the world, interact with the world, and live in the world is challenging and requires ongoing commitment. It ain't easy, but it is possible. One of the biggest things that gets in the way is our inner judge, who is always telling us that we are not smart enough, thin enough, fit enough, rich enough, able enough, or worthy enough to live our dreams. If we believe the judge, we sentence ourselves to something less than ideal, something almost good enough, something inferior. We settle for a vanilla life and a vanilla mind-set while longing for a chocolate life with hot fudge and sprinkles. Setting aside the habit of self judging is a step toward living the life you want.

The problem with self judgment is that we usually judge ourselves too harshly. I have met people who have the opposite problem—judging themselves as near perfect gifts to the world. Most of us, however, decree to ourselves that we are lacking, substandard, inferior, and second-rate human beings. As I pause for just a second to listen to my inner judge, I hear that I am a failure who is too short, a bad speller, twenty-five pounds overweight, uncreative, lazy, willful, and stubborn.

Try it yourself. Close your eyes and take a few long, deep breaths. Now bring an image of your inner judge to mind. Listen for your judge's voice, and use the space provided to jot down what you hear.

_____

_____

_____

_____

_____

Do you judge yourself as harshly as I judge myself? Odds are you do. For years my inner judge reigned. He spouted off constantly about everything I did wrong (and *everything* I did was wrong). He belittled my dreams, he sabotaged my efforts to change, and he chattered until he had me second-guessing my every decision. As I have worked to change my mind-set, I have taken steps to cut down on the power my inner judge has over me. I have not figured out how to stop him completely, but I have managed to take away a lot of the power he used to hold. Three tactics have helped me get ahead of the judge: staying in the present, catching the judge at work, and asking myself if the judgment is true.

STAYING IN THE PRESENT

The more you are able to stop living in the past or the future and focus your mind on living right now in this moment, the less self judging you do. Our inner judges are much more vocal when we are worrying about the past and fretting about the future. Of course, staying in the present is no easy task if your mind is used to fluttering through time and space. Awareness is the key.

One option is to catch your mind wandering. When you realize you have started thinking about something else when you are trying to be in the moment with a special person—how you really need to clean the refrigerator later to track down that odd smell, or contemplating hairstyles of the late 1980s—gently redirect your mind back to that special person. Don't scold yourself, just nudge your mind back to the present.

Another option is to make as much eye contact as possible with the person with whom you are interacting. It is harder for your mind to skip around the past and the future when your eyes are locked on someone in the here and now.

CATCHING YOUR INNER JUDGE AT WORK

Simply being aware that you are judging yourself is often enough to stop it from happening. When I catch my inner judge at work, I simply take a few breaths, let my head clear, and move on with my day. Catching your inner judge takes practice, but if you pay attention, you will succeed. You may hear your judge as a voice in your head, you may feel it as a tightness in your chest, or it may manifest itself as a generally uncomfortable feeling from head to toe. You have to get a feel for how your judge makes itself known. At first, it might be challenging, but the more you practice, the easier it becomes.

ASKING YOURSELF IF THE JUDGMENT IS TRUE

If your inner judge makes a statement that is not true, call him on it. For example, my inner judge says I am lazy. I don't agree. The problem here is that my inner judge confuses resting with laziness. My judge knows that I want to accomplish a lot of things during my dash, and when he sees me resting he thinks I'm being lazy. Every time I hear the "you're lazy" judgment rattling around in my head, I counter it by mentally reciting my schedule or recent accomplishments. This makes him back off a bit.

Evaluating Your Inner Judge

What about when a judgment is accurate? In my situation, I am a horrible speller, and it would be good to lose twenty-five pounds or so. In these cases, I acknowledge that my inner judge is right, and then make a statement to myself like, "I am a bad speller, but that does not define me. I'm a lot better than I used to be, my computer catches most of my mistakes, and proofreaders catch most of the others" or, "I do have some more weight to lose, but I am eating healthier and exercising more than I used to. I have also managed to keep off the weight I lost last year." If a new self judgment pops into my head that has some truth to it, I literally make a note of it and then devote some time to that judgment the next time I meditate. This usually helps me figure out a way to address the issue in a healthy manner.

While we tend to judge ourselves harshly, self judgment isn't good or bad, it just is. Your self judgments may be irrational, or they may be full of truth; they may hinder progress, or they may be useful in determining where you need to make progress. The important thing is not allowing your inner judge to control your daily experience.

DECISIONOMETER

It is harder for most people to make a decision than it is for them to live with the decision once made. They fret, fidget, fuss, flip, flop, fiddle, and bubble over decisions. They second-, triple-, and quadruple-guess themselves, putting even simple decisions off until the last minute. The fact is that most decisions are not worth this much attention.

The deceptively simple-looking Decisionometer can help. It resembles a standard issue U.S. quarter. It is, in fact, outwardly identical to a quarter. Just toss it into the air to activate its decision-making microprocessor. While it is falling, state the pending decision in the form of a yes or no question. The Decisionometer makes your decision for you when it hits the floor: heads equals yes, tails equals no. With the decision made, you can move on with your life and use all the time you would have spent floundering, worrying, and stewing about the decision to do something nice for yourself. The Decisionometer retails for $19.95 and is worth every penny.

How Is Your Balance?

I think one of the biggest things hindering a healthy mind-set in most people is lack of balance in their lives. It is easy to gravitate to extremes. I didn't plan to gain those twenty-five pounds my inner judge harps at me about. It happened slowly, over time. I let my diet get out of balance by eating more calories than I burned. I was not being mindful about eating appropriately.

Many caregivers I have met have a difficult time balancing their work life and their home life. Many others struggle to balance time invested in the care of others and time invested in their own care. In most situations, life is most fulfilling when we can exist in the happy middle. I have worked hard to balance my calories in and calories out so that I am no longer gaining weight, and I look at that as a small victory. The next step in my search for equilibrium is better balancing the time I spend sitting in front of the television and the time I spend on my bike or treadmill. If I get up and get moving more I can melt away those twenty-five extra pounds. Balance and mind-set are tied to each other. Paying attention to your mind-set gives you a feeling for your balance. When you are more self-aware, you are better able to sense when emotions, relationships, and other parts of your life are out of balance. On the other hand, if a part of your life is way out of balance, it is very difficult to pay attention to your mind-set.

The lack of balance leaves you feeling cluttered and foggy, which makes knowing your own mind difficult. Sometime we have to push ourselves; balance is not easy, but it is doable. We can train ourselves to make the changes we need in our lives. Before you read any further, spend a few minutes sitting with your eyes closed thinking about different areas of your life (work, home, relationships, health, diet, and so forth) and get a feel for how your balance is in each area. Just taking the time to give the topic some thought is a step toward better understanding your balance. In chapter 7, I discuss the concept of balance in more depth.

Do You See Your Options?

At a recent event, an acquaintance who attended a daylong presentation I gave graciously complimented me. She was very kind and her words seemed sincere. We have known each other for years, and I thought we had a positive and friendly relationship. Then, within twenty-four hours of the session's end, I heard from two people (independent of each other) how this acquaintance was overheard talking negatively about my presentation and me. What was going on here? In my mind, there were a few possibilities:

1. My acquaintance was misheard or misunderstood.
2. My acquaintance was saying one thing to my face and other things behind my back.
3. The two individuals were (consciously or unconsciously) trying to drive a wedge between my acquaintance and me.
4. My acquaintance didn't like my presentation but did not want to hurt my feelings by saying so.

I also saw a few options for dealing with the situation:

A. I could confront my acquaintance and ask her what was going on.
B. I could fret and worry and stress over it, but not say a word.
C. I could let it go and move on with my life.
D. I could start talking about her behind her back.

I chose C. I let it go and moved on with my life.

There was a time in my life when I would not have even seen that as an option. The truth is, I would have gravitated toward A, B, and D. I would have gone to my hotel room and fretted all night, confronted her in the morning, and depending on the outcome of that conversation I might have started a whisper campaign about her. I'm not proud that I was like that, but it is who I was. All too often my problem was that I reacted to situations without considering my options. I acted before thinking or, maybe, I acted without thinking at all. As I work to change my mind-set, I make it a point to spend more time thinking about my options. Here are some questions to consider:

When and how do you respond to situations automatically?

_____

_____

_____

When do you stop to consider your options when confronted with troubling situations? What makes it easier to do this in some situations than in others?

_____

_____

_____

What kinds of options are the easiest for you to see? What kinds of options are harder? What patterns are revealed when you think about these options?

_____

_____

_____

While it is a good idea to consider your options, I don't want you to agonize over making a decision. After considering all your options, trust your gut and go with the one that you feel is right.

What Else Can You Do to Mend Your Mind-Set?

Rewiring your thinking is not easy, partially because you are the only one who can do the work, and you are the only one who can really decide what changes you need to make. Others can suggest, badger, hint, propose, imply, and recommend, but nothing happens until you decide to make a change and then take some sort of action. If I had not been open and ready for change everything my friend Chris had to say would have gone in one ear and out the other.

I'm assuming that since you have read this far you are at least a bit receptive to ideas for change. The remainder of this chapter looks at mind-set adjustments you might want to consider. Make the most of ideas that speak to you right now, and note things you may want to think more about later. If you're not ready to make changes right now, you can always fold the corner of this page and come back to it when you are ready.

LET IT GO

Chris was fond of telling the following story to students in his tae kwon do and yoga classes.

> There were once two young monks from a very strict monastic order traveling through the countryside. They had both recently taken vows of silence and chastity. They had sworn to remain silent and not think about, look at, or touch women. As they traveled through the forest, they came upon a beautiful young maiden standing nervously next to a roaring stream. The first monk diverted his eyes and gingerly crossed the stream. Without a word, the second monk gracefully picked up the young woman, carried her across the raging stream, and put her down high and dry on the opposite shore.
>
> The first monk glared red-faced and angry at his traveling companion as they walked on. Hours passed. The first monk's anger did not dissipate. In fact, it increased. His face tightened. Steam shot from his ears. His footsteps pounded the path.
>
> That night they camped under the stars. The second monk slept soundly. Consumed with anger, the first monk slept fitfully.

In fact, he did not sleep well for the next week nor did his irritation with his companion decrease.

After seven days of silent rage he could stand it no longer. As they approached the gates to their monastery, he yelled, "Brother Monk, you broke your most sacred vows when you touched that woman! How could you! Do you not respect the teachings of our religion? How can you return to the monastery after desecrating our beliefs?"

The second monk stopped for a moment before passing through the gates and whispered, "Brother, I left the woman at the stream. Why have you been carrying her for a week?"

Which monk are you most like? Do you carry things around, letting them eat at you until you burst, or do you let go and move on with life? If you do hold on to things and constantly hear them rattling, clattering, and clanging around in your head, consider the following questions:

What does holding on to the things I carry around give me?

_____

_____

_____

How does holding on to things affect my relationships, career, sleep, and attitude?

_____

_____

_____

Where did my habit of hanging on come from? Why?

_____

_____

_____

What would happen if I let some things go?

_____

_____

_____

NO ONE IS PERFECT

Perfection is a myth. We may think we see it in people we want to emulate, we may expect it of ourselves, others may expect it from us, we may expect it from others, but it just does not exist. I went to school with a girl who had an emotional meltdown after receiving her lowest grade ever—an A-. She was so wrapped up in the idea that she was a perfect student that realizing she wasn't shook her to her core. It is hard to erase the image of her hyperventilating and throwing up on the floor. It was a long time ago, but I still remember the diced carrots.

There is nothing wrong with striving for perfection, but I think we should also temper those efforts with the realization that our labors are going to fall short of that lofty goal. I am not advocating we lower our standards or quit improving. I am not suggesting we accept or expect anything but the best from ourselves. What I am saying is we need to accept "acceptable" willingly when our efforts at perfection fail, because we are not infallible. If you find yourself trapped in the myth of perfection, consider the following questions:

How did you acquire your need for perfection?

_____

_____

_____

What does being a perfectionist get you? How does it make your life better?

_____

_____

_____

Where in your life does perfectionism get in the way? Why?

_____

_____

_____

What would happen if you settled for "good enough"?

_____

_____

_____

SAY "YES" TO YOURSELF

Many caregivers have a mind-set that says, "Do for others. Take care of others. Invest time, energy, and resources in others." These individuals have a hard time saying "yes" to meeting their own needs because meeting the needs of the people around them is so consuming. They are devoted to the welfare and happiness of others, but are unable to say yes to meeting their own needs.

You may want to candidly consider investing some of your resources in your own well-being. Learning to be kind to yourself is hard when you are used to putting yourself last. Upon reflection, you may realize you have no history of being kind to yourself as an adult. You might not know how to say "yes" to meeting your own needs. If you can say "yes" to meeting your needs, chances are you probably don't do it enough, or you feel guilty for being so selfish. I mean, how dare you think you should be able to spend half an hour enjoying some "me time!" Learning to say "yes" to yourself makes you happier and healthier, and it makes you better at taking care of all the people you nurture in your life.

We get in the habit of self-denial, self-sacrifice, and self-deprecation and then wonder why we feel so miserable. We work long hours, take on more and more projects and responsibilities, push ourselves further and further, and find saying "no" to requests for our time and talent difficult. We literally give until it hurts—sometimes physically, sometimes emotionally. Fixing this "yes to everyone but me" attitude boils down to giving yourself what you need when you need it.

Here is another tale Chris shared with his students.

> A student once asked his teacher, "Master, what is enlightenment?"
>
> The master replied, "When hungry, eat. When tired, sleep."

Are you enlightened? Do you eat when hungry and sleep when tired, or do you deny yourself what you need when you need it?

Speaking of needs, what do you need right now in this very moment? Do you need a foot massage? Do you need a hunk of cheesecake? Do you need a kind word or two from your sweetie? Do you need to walk barefoot through dewy grass as the sun rises after a wild night out? Do you need a nap? Do you need three minutes alone in a quiet room? Do you need to scream? Do you need to feel your toes curl and your breath catch in your throat?

I know you may not be able to drop this book and go get what you need at this very moment, so I am not going to suggest it. What I am suggesting is that you spend some time thinking about something you need—something simple and doable, something frivolous, something out of *your* ordinary—and then make it happen in the next forty-eight hours. You can address big issues later; right now, you need to practice caring for yourself. You need to practice *not* denying yourself what you need when you need it.

FIND FREEDOM *IN* EMOTIONS

I spent years—no, make that decades—of my life hiding from my emotions. I ignored them, hid from them, and pretended I did not have them. I swallowed them, repressed them, and crammed them into the dark, cobwebby corners of my mind. It did not work, of course. From time to time, they would burst through my chest, spew out my mouth, or blow off the top of my head. I thought this was a "guy thing" when I was young. I thought real men just did not let their emotions show. Case closed. After twenty plus years working in a female dominated profession, I know differently. I know that many, many women handle their emotions exactly the same way.

As a nation, it seems we are afraid to feel. It seems we think we need to be above our emotions. It seems we would prefer a life without the messiness and unpredictability of feelings. I see this in twenty-somethings just starting out in the world and in baby boomers who came of age in the love-and-peace and get-in-touch-with-your-inner-self days of the late sixties and early seventies. I am not smart enough to understand why this is the case, but I see it all over the country when I speak to caregivers.

The mind-set change I encourage you to consider involves learning to find freedom *in* your emotions instead of trying to find freedom *from* your emotions. This does not have to be a complicated undertaking. Just give yourself permission to feel what you are feeling in any given moment. Acknowledge your feelings, feel them, and then let them go.

I used to get terribly angry with all the bad drivers on the road. I swallowed that anger, tried to suppress it, until I could hold it in no longer. Then my driving would become overly aggressive, I would yell and flip off the "bad" drivers, and I'd feel like I was having a stroke by the time I completed my one-mile commute.

If you picture me in the above paragraph, you might conclude I was feeling my emotions. I was reacting very emotionally—I was angry, enraged, ticked off—but it did not have much to do with the other drivers. These outbursts had more to do with the work-related feelings I was suppressing. At the end of the day, I was taking out on my fellow drivers the frustrations, disappointments, and anger I suppressed all day long at work.

As I have made feeling my emotions in the moment, as they come to me, a habit, my road rage has dissipated. I don't blow up anymore. That throbbing vein in my forehead is no longer at risk of bursting. When something disappoints me, I spend a few moments being disappointed. When something makes me happy, I allow myself to enjoy that happiness. When I am hurt, I feel hurt. Life is more fulfilling this way, I feel more in tune, more complete, more fulfilled.

Allowing yourself to feel your emotions instead of ignoring them is not easy, but if you can change this mind-set, you can change your life. As you go through the next day of your life, make an effort to name your feelings as you experience them. What are you feeling when you hit the snooze button for the third time? What are you feeling when you get your first hug of the day? What are you feeling when your sweetie comes home from work? Once you name a feeling, give yourself a moment or two (or more) to feel it before moving on with your day.

CHANGE YOUR SPACE TO CHANGE YOUR MIND

Our environments influence our mind-sets. It is easier to eat healthily when you stock your house with healthy food choices instead of wall-to-wall cake, cookies, and empty calories. It is easier to say "yes" to yourself when the people around you support your decision to invest time and energy in your well-being. It is easier to feel your emotions as they come when your environment is safe, nurturing, and supportive.

With this in mind, I encourage you to step back, look at both your physical and emotional environments, and write down your thoughts about the following questions:

What aspects of the physical environments you inhabit every day make living your Ultimate Purpose a challenge?

_____

_____

_____

_____

What three things about your physical environment can you change to help improve your mind-set?

_____

_____

_____

What aspects of the emotional environments you inhabit every day make living your Ultimate Purpose a challenge?

_____

_____

_____

What three things about your emotional environment can you change to help improve your mind-set?

_____

_____

_____

You'll probably find it impossible to wholly remake both your physical and emotional environments all at once, but you don't have to. It's okay to start with small changes. They can lead to big results. When I decided to stop thinking about writing and start writing, the first thing I had to do was find the top of my desk. It was nearly impossible to write until I could find my computer and a little bit of clear desktop. It was a small step, and it led to other, larger steps. That clear desktop became an oasis. You might want to consider creating an oasis for yourself at home or work—a small space where you can clear your head, focus, and get to work on living.

GIVE PARENTS A BREAK

Over the last few years, I've heard repeatedly from early care and education professionals across the country that parents are one of the biggest causes of caregiver stress. I regularly hear that parents do not pay their bills on time. I hear they do not "get it" when it comes to rearing their children. I hear they are disrespectful. I hear they do not really care about their children. I hear they are unappreciative. I hear they take their caregivers for granted. I hear they are more concerned with their jobs and their stuff than they are with their children. And I hear specifics that are much, much worse.

I think many providers use these complaints as a way to vent their own stress; it is incredibly human to feel better about yourself by pointing out someone else's shortcomings. It is also easier to point out another person's flaws than it is to examine your own. I think most caregivers need to take a step back and give parents a break.

On top of that, we seldom see parents at their best. We see them at the mercy of their hectic schedules. We see them rushing to work in the morning or at the end of the day when they are tired, stressed, and beaten by the day. We see them struggling to leave their infants, flummoxed by their fitful toddlers, puzzled by their preschoolers' erratic sleep habits, or vexed by their school-agers' recent spelling test performances. We see parents overwhelmed by their jobs, their class schedules, their personal lives, their finances, their car troubles, their sick cat, their aching backs, or all of the above.

What's more, we are not always at *our* best when we see them. Drop-off and pickup times, those tough transition periods that bookend our days, are often hurried times when no one is operating at their best. Because of multiple comings and goings, we are frequently unable to give each parent the attention they may want and need. We are unable to invest the time needed for good communication, empathy, and emotional connection. On top of all this, there is also a chance that we are tired, tense, lethargic, anxious, or agitated by the stress of our work or personal lives.

Don't get me wrong, I have had the displeasure of working with some truly horrible parents—parents who did not deserve the wonderful children they were blessed with and who were not doing right by those children. I understand that there are bad parents out there.

The parents I want you to give a break are the average mommies and daddies, the parents who are struggling to make it through the day just like you, the parents who want the best for their child but are unsure what "the best" looks like, the parents who, like all of us, are too often overburdened with the rush of life. Give a break to the parents who are doing the best they can for their children with the resources available to them.

It would be wrong of me to suggest you give parents a break without offering some helpful suggestions:

- Be mindful of your feelings: Know how you allow your feelings to influence your reactions to the parents with whom you work.

- Avoid getting on their emotional rollercoaster: Don't allow the feelings, experiences, worries, and thoughts parents share overwhelm you. Empathy is part of our job, but internalizing the emotions of others is harmful.

- Control your stress: Our stress has influence over our reaction to other people *and* their reaction to us. Keeping your stress in check affects everyone you meet in a positive way.

- Let go of the little stuff: Sometimes we let one little comment, expression, or perceived slight ruin our whole day. Letting go of these things—not allowing them to clutter our minds and control our days—makes our lives less stressful.

- Remember who is in control: You may not be able to control the people you come in contact with, but you are always in control of your reaction to them.

- Offer the benefit of the doubt: Always assume that parents are acting with good intentions and in the best interest of their families.

- Know that you do not know it all: Our limited contact with parents is usually not enough for us to know what is really happening in their lives. Realize you only see a small snapshot of who they are during a hurried part of the day.

- Be available to support them as much as you are able: Know your limits. Make sure they know that you have limits. Know when to say "no" and then be strong enough to say it.

If you have children of your own or if you have ever been a child, you can imagine how stressful and challenging the job is. Most parents are working hard to make good choices, provide proper guidance, create nurturing environments, be positive role models, and do all the things good parents do for their children. Give them a break.

Remember that no matter how bad you might think they are, *they were smart enough to choose you as their child's caregiver.*

Tactics, Tools, and Tips

1. It is important to open yourself to new ideas and experiences as you begin to change your mind-set. You do not want to continue missing opportunities that your old mind-sets were preventing you from seeing. You don't want to overlook something that may bring you closer to living your Ultimate Purpose. I suggest that you purchase a small pocket notebook, and keep it and a pen with you at all times. Use these tools to collect ideas, goals, dreams, feelings, observations, concerns, insights, and musings as you move through your day. It is a good idea to include the date for future reference. This not only keeps you from missing important things that pop into your head, it also helps keep you focused on your efforts to keep your smile for the long haul, and the constant attention to your thinking makes changing your habits easier.

   As you add things to your notebook, periodically make time to review and organize them. Do you see recurring themes and ideas? Are certain topics always popping into your head? Do you see patterns in your thinking that you want to understand better? As your self-understanding grows, make sure you do something with your insights.

2. Now that you have spent some time thinking about your Ultimate Purpose and considering changes to your mind-set, actively seek out people who share your goals and dreams, who can help guide you where you want to go, and who shine with a passion you want to emulate. Building a network of such people provides a system that positively influences your efforts, guides you along your path, smooths out road bumps, and offers all kinds of valuable support.

   In my experience, these role models and mentors kind of just appear when you need them. You just have to be on the lookout so you do not miss them when they pop up. When you take your head out of the sand and open your eyes, you see that the world is full of people ready to lend a helping hand on your life journey. My buddy Chris was a big supporter during the early days of my transformation, and there were many others. The more I open myself up to the idea of growth, the more needed supporters and cheerleaders appear to help me move forward.

If the mentors, supporters, and cheerleaders you need don't seem to be popping up in front of your eyes, consider joining clubs, groups, and other organizations related to your professional or personal interests. Put yourself in situations where contact with the people you need in your life is most likely, and then work to build real and honest relationships with those people. As you grow into the person you want to be, it is important to remember to give back by being available to help others on their journey.

Chris gave me a lot, and I try to never miss a chance to pay him back by sharing what he taught me.

Six

Enriching
Your Environments

AWARENESS OF OUR MORTALITY is important because it can galvanize us to make the most of our life. Knowing that our time is limited can be a scary thing, but it can also encourage us to get busy living. Remember that in the end your life is summed up by a little dash separating the year you were born and the year you died—make the most of it. We need to know our days are numbered and then live each of those days with the intellectual curiosity, freshness, and joy of an infant or toddler. As with infants and toddlers, the physical and emotional environments we live in play a major role in our overall happiness. It is difficult to be happy and fulfilled if the spaces, people, and relationships around us don't provide what we need. With that in mind, we're going to look at the beginning of someone's life and see what we can glean from her environment that will help us make ours better.

Annie's love-worn, stuffed pink elephant observes from atop the piano as she glues her eyes to the side of the aquarium to watch as our Red-Eared Slider turtle eviscerates a dead Dalmatian Molly fish Tasha has fed him. The turtle methodically chomps away on his breakfast as the curious two-year-old watches wide-eyed. After a few moments, she turns her attention back to a tote full of plastic dinosaurs. She carefully lines up a triceratops family, a mommy and three sisters. She shows me the smallest of the four and says, "It's me!"

Her attention turns again, this time to Siddha, who passes by wearing a blanket as a cape. Annie heads off to put on her own cape, but as soon as she gets it on, she decides she has to go potty. Off comes the cape, and she races for the bathroom door. A few minutes later, she emerges with a smile and tells me she remembered to wash her hands. She bypasses her abandoned cape and speeds, on tiptoes, to breakfast. I ask if she would like to eat a dead fish for breakfast like the turtle. She nods her head with a mischievous smile.

Breakfast is over. Now Annie is wearing a fuzzy pink back-pack full of board books and some pink slippers. Her arms are full of more books. She chatters as she climbs into her car—a long toy box—and shouts, "Siddha, come on! Get your seat belt on! Get your shoes on! It's school bus time! It's all right! That's fine!" Siddha crawls in behind Annie and they drive off.

Annie has added a purse and a blue hat to her slippers and backpack. Her bags and arms are weighed down with books. She can barely walk. School is over, and so they climb back into the toy box car and head to the library. They talk and argue and bicker and chitter like happy squirrels. They express them-selves with body language as much as with words—rolling their eyes, pointing fingers, tossing back heads, and stomping their feet.

I don't catch all that Siddha and Annie have to say, but I hear bits of conversation about our walk yesterday. They talk about the two cats we saw at the flower shop, the purple ceiling at the coffee shop, the loud machine that was "breaking the street," and the scary garbage truck. Their whole morning ends up being one long evolving dramatic play scenario full of words and feelings and thinking and creativity and problem-solving and learning.

Annie and Siddha have been part of our family child care since they were a few weeks old. We have worked hard to create an emotional and physical environment that nurtures them and meets their ever-changing needs.

What we have done for Annie and Siddha is not special or unusual. Professional child care providers all over the world work hard to make sure their programs offer physical and emo-tional spaces that are conducive to early care and learning. They read books, attend trainings, keep up-to-date on the latest research, and spend lots of time evaluating their successes and failures. Sadly, they generally do not devote nearly as much attention to the kinds of environments they create for themselves.

Caregivers need to devote time to building quality physical and emotional environments for themselves, because no one else is going to do it for them. We need to put as much thought into the spaces we create for ourselves as we put into the ones we create for children. Tasha and I put lots of effort into creating an environment where Annie and Siddha can play with comfort and ease, an environment that is responsive, engaging, nurturing, fresh, joyful, and full of intellectual stimulation. The quality of the physical and emotional environments we have built for ourselves has also received plenty of time and energy because it is just as important to our success as caregivers. If we do not live in nurturing environments, it is difficult to create those environments for children.

Children are not the only ones who deserve environments that nurture them as individuals—environments that are warm, inviting, and safe. Sadly, too many people—children and adults—spend their days surrounded by strife, chaos, and clutter. We all deserve environments that allow us to be the best we can be. You are probably working very hard and burning lots of time and energy assuring the environments you create for children are strong and healthy. Now I want you to spend time considering the environments you create for yourself.

Throughout the rest of this chapter, I want you to consider some questions about your personal physical and emotional environments. The goal is to get you to think about doing for yourself some of the things you do for children, to get you to invest in your own physical and emotional environments. No one else is going to take responsibility for making your surroundings better. You have to do it yourself.

YOUTUNES

Ever wish your life came equipped with a soundtrack? You know, music and sound effects that depict your thoughts and feelings as you move through your day, letting others know what to expect when they encounter you, and filling you with courage or calm when needed. Well, for a monthly subscription of just $9.95 you can subscribe to YouTunes and receive music to live by.

The perfect song or sound for every situation automatically fills your environment as soon as our neural implants and environmental sensors detect your musical needs. In the olden days, YouTunes was simply a really empathetic dude following you around holding a large boom box over his head. He adjusted the volume as needed and stopped to change the cassette tape when he sensed a change in your musical needs. Now, thanks to digital media and nanotechnology, YouTunes can sense what you are thinking and provide the needed background music through a series of hovering speakers made invisible through the same technology used in the Cloak of Tranquility.

Order now and we'll throw in 1,500 top-rated cartoon sound effects that will make you love slipping on banana peels and falling off cliffs while holding anvils.

Do Your Environments Feel Safe and Inviting?

Annie and Siddha are able to play so well together in our program because we have created a space for them that is both physically and emotionally safe. They know what to expect. Because they feel safe, they are secure enough to take learning risks. This was evident on the walk they were discussing during their play. When approached by the cats in the flower shop, when they saw the skid loader breaking up a section of concrete in the street, and when the garbage truck roared up, they both automatically looked to me. In each of those situations, I caught their gaze and assured them that they were safe and that nothing was going to hurt them. That assurance allowed them to relax and enjoy the new experiences.

We know that little minds crave new experiences, and we work hard to provide them. This makes our program inviting. It might be friendly flower shop cats or a hungry turtle, but we work to ensure the children in our care find inviting ideas, materials, and experiences every day. Take some time to consider the following questions:

In what ways do your physical environments feel safe?

_____

_____

_____

In what ways do they feel unsafe?

_____

_____

_____

In what ways do the people and relationships in your life create safety for you?

_____

_____

_____

In what ways do they cause you stress, anxiety, strife, or fear?

_____

_____

_____

What two things could you change in your emotional environment to make it feel safer?

_____

_____

_____

_____

What two things could you change in your physical environment to make it feel safer?

_____

_____

_____

_____

How does your physical surrounding offer you new experiences, encourage you to try new things, or support you in taking risks?

_____

_____

_____

_____

How do the people and relationships in your life offer you new experiences, encourage you to try new things, or support you in taking risks?

_____

_____

_____

_____

Are Your Environments Well Organized?

Tasha and I organize our environment to ensure Annie and Siddha can find the props and tools they need to facilitate their exploration of the world. This organization includes the emotional environment. They are able to predict what kind of responses they will get from us and that they will get the nurturing and affection they need when they need it. This is important. Living in a disorganized and unpredictable emotional environment can be troubling for children and adults. In my experience, the more organized I am, the more effective I am. I used to hide from life under piles of papers and mountains of emotional clutter. As I have weeded through this mess, I have found a more fulfilling life.

Consider the physical and emotional environments you live in for a few minutes. Are they organized in a way that is conducive to healthy living? I once met a center director who told me about a piece of her physical environment that was really letting her down and making life tough. Her husband had remodeled the bathroom at their house. It was beautiful. She loved it. It had turned out just the way she wanted it, except that her husband had not installed the last few pieces of the sink drain. This meant she had to use the sink in the kitchen. A few days of this would not have bothered her, but it had been like this for over six months. They had gotten used to living without a functioning bathroom sink, but when she thought about it, she experienced all the emotions you are imagining she experienced.

We all have things like this in our lives—things that are not ideal that we get used to over time. Some are bigger, some smaller, and they all make our environments just a little more challenging. Are you putting as much time and energy into your own environments as you are putting into the environments you create for others? Our physical and emotional surroundings play a huge part in how our lives unfold. Spending some time contemplating yours is a good idea:

How does the organization of your physical surroundings support your daily life?

In what ways does physical disorganization get in your way?

What things are most "right" about your physical and emotional environments?

_____

_____

_____

In what ways are the people and relationships in your life predictable and nurturing?

_____

_____

_____

In what ways are they unpredictable or distressing?

_____

_____

_____

What three steps can you take to make your environments a little more organized and predictable?

_____

_____

_____

Grab some paper and sketch a room from your personal physical environment as you would like it to look. Next, draw two pictures of your emotional environment—one as it looks right now and another as you would like it to look in six months. What are the differences between the two pictures?

When it comes to altering your environments, taking baby steps is the way to go. Trying to change too much too quickly can be overwhelming and lead to more problems. You have to also remember to nurture the parts of your environments that are healthy and bring you joy. We tend to ignore these things, or completely forget them, when life gets hectic and hard. You will find that making improvements to your physical environments leads to healthier emotional environments, so that might be a good place to start. Life is just easier if you can consistently find your car keys and don't have to use the kitchen sink to brush your teeth. If you need some help with your physical environment, check out www.flylady.net. I know many caregivers who have made their lives better with ideas they found on that Web site.

Do You Have Routines?

Routines are another way we organize our family child care environment. The children in our program know we pick up toys and wash our hands before lunch and we read stories after lunch before taking rests. Simple routines bring order and make life predictable for the children. This makes them feel safe and helps them maneuver through their day.

I find that routines make my life flow a bit easier too. I like a cup of chai tea in the morning after I do yoga and meditation and before the children start arriving. When I am on the road, I like to order Chinese takeout the night before I present. If I have to be away overnight, I leave Tasha a love letter on her nightstand before I leave.

Sometimes, however, routines bring more nuisances than flow to our lives. We become overwhelmed with little things like remembering to put out the garbage and recycling on Sunday night, getting the cable bill paid by the 21st, and sanitizing the changing table for the 14th time in one day. These things are unavoidable potholes in the road of life—ugly necessities. The best way I have found to deal with them is to change my mind-set. Instead of seeing them as unwelcome hindrances to the flow of my life, I see them as important pieces of the bigger picture. If I want an uncluttered living space that does not smell like rotten diapers and decomposing kitchen waste, I need to take out the trash. If I want to unwind at the end of the day with a rerun of *Law & Order,* I have to pay the cable bill. If I want everyone to stay healthy, I have to clean the changing table. This mind-set toward the mundane, must-do parts of life makes things easier to tolerate. I mark them off my mental checklist with a smile, knowing I have accomplished something important.

While some routines can make us feel safe and secure, others are the causes of our stress. Some people have a hard time with routines like their commute to work, unproductive meetings, and repetitive tasks like diaper changing. Here are some ways to gain understanding of your good and bad routines:

Make a list of routines in your life that cause you stress, tension, frustration, or anger.

Make a list of routines in your life that are not physically or emotionally healthy.

Consider the lists you just made and then use the space provided to hatch an ingenious plan to rid your life of your hurtful routines. If your plan requires you to fly backwards around the earth real fast to reverse the flow of time like Superman did when Lois Lane died in the 1978 *Superman* or requires you to change the future by sending a robot bodyguard into the past like in the 1984 *The Terminator,* go right ahead. Make a plan that gets the job done.

Make a list of routines in your life that make you feel happy, safe, and fulfilled.

List three new routines that would make your life better if you implemented them.

_____

_____

_____

Do Your Environments Avoid Overstimulation?

Child care environments need to offer enough stimulation to engage young minds, but not so much that those young minds overheat. Too much stimulation can be as bad as not enough stimulation. Balance is important.

We adults have to think about how much stimulation our own minds are getting from the environments we create for ourselves. Many of us tend to gravitate toward overstimulation. We take on lots of projects, try to multitask, and cope not only with our emotional baggage but also with the emotional baggage of the people around us. Overstimulated infants shut down and go to sleep to give their minds a chance to reset, but many overstimulated adults grab another cup of coffee or an energy drink.

I think many of us overstimulate ourselves because it keeps our minds busy. When we are busy thinking about all our worldly projects and activities, we can avoid thinking about our darkness and inner turmoil.

I recently realized that for the first year after my dad died of lung cancer I kept myself overly busy to avoid thinking about the loss. It was painful to address all the emotions that bubbled up when I thought about his passing. So I did everything I could not to think about it. That was not particularly healthy either. The truth is the best thing we can do to address our darkness and inner turmoil is to admit they exist and are part of us. Doing so helped me slow down and stop working so hard to hide from those feelings. I still miss my father, but it does not hurt to think about him. I am no longer overtaxing, overextending, and overstimulating myself trying to hide from the reality of his death.

If you want to slow down and stop overworking yourself, you may need to consider what is driving you to push yourself so hard. Is there something you need to address? Is there part of your life you need to stop hiding from and just accept? Take some time and answer these questions:

What three things could you cut from your environments to reduce overstimulation?

_____

_____

_____

Do you use frenetic busyness to protect yourself from dealing with inner demons and emotional baggage? If so, why?

_____

_____

_____

Write about a time when you felt overwhelmed by life.

_____

_____

_____

What steps can you take in your life to prevent things like what you described above?

_____

_____

_____

Are Your Environments Nurturing?

As I have said before, caregivers are good at nurturing the people around them, but generally bad at nurturing themselves. We devote so much time to others that we don't believe we have the time or energy to nurture our own needs. We feel guilty taking care of ourselves—we feel we are being selfish. I think many of us also see needing to nurture ourselves as a sign of weakness.

If we are to nurture others successfully over the long term, we need to nurture ourselves. Investing time and energy in self-care gives us a wide and deep foundation for all we do for other people. Gustav is a good example. He's a guy I know who has worked for nearly forty years administering programs that serve children and families. His work has made life better for thousands of families over the years, and it reaches all corners of his community. A little over ten years ago, Gustav went through a stretch where he was not caring for himself very well or very consistently; for the most part, he had been good at nurturing his own needs. Gustav is only one of many long-term caregivers I have met over the years who have devoted thirty, forty, or up to fifty years serving others as their career. Some have cared for multiple generations of the same family. Most have some hard times along the way, but generally have long, quiet careers devoted to nurturing children. Sadly, our profession loses many caregivers who feel the same devotion but never find a way to meet their own needs.

Use the following activities to help build a more nurturing environment for yourself:

Write down one thing you could do right now that would feel good or bring you joy, peace, or relaxation.

_____

_____

Put this book down right now and go do that one thing. When you come back, use the space provided to describe how you felt doing that activity.

_____

_____

_____

_____

Make a list of four people in your life who do the most to nurture you and your dreams, goals, and happiness. By each name, write why the person is so supportive.

_____

_____

_____

_____

The people you listed are your supporters and cheerleaders. Make it a point to find some unhurried time to spend with them this week.

In the following space, list twenty other things you can do that would feel good or bring you joy, relaxation, or peace. Commit to doing at least one of them every week.

_____

_____

_____

_____

_____

_____

_____

_____

Do Your Environments Focus on Healthy Choices?

As caregivers we spend a lot of time promoting healthy life habits to children, but not all of us take the advice we dish out. We tell kids to eat healthy, but we do not. We tell kids to get enough sleep, but we do not. We tell kids to exercise, but we do not. We tell kids to make good choices, but we do not. We tell kids to think before they act, but we do not.

Life is simply better when you are emotionally and physically healthy. Practicing the things we preach to the children in our own lives goes a long way in helping us maintain our smiles. It is much easier to tell others what is good for them than it is to take our own advice. I am always struggling with the choices I make about things such as television, food, exercise, and balancing work life and home life. It is easier for me to advocate for healthy choices than it is to make those choices consistently. I'm sure you have the same struggles in your own life. The point is our lives are better when we win these difficult struggles, and we can win. I've won a few myself and know many providers who have improved their lives immensely by making changes to the way they approach their lives.

Use the questions that follow to help you better understand the health-related choices you are making.

What two changes could you make to live a healthier life?

_____

_____

What is holding you back from making those changes?

_____

_____

_____

What scares you about making these changes?

_____

_____

What one step can you take to begin forming new, healthier habits?

_____

_____

Do Your Environments Encourage Curiosity, Self-Awareness, and Personal Growth?

Are you putting as much effort into your own cognitive development as you are putting into the cognitive development of the children you care for? We know young children's healthy development depends on feeding their little minds, but we wrongfully assume our brains are completely developed once we reach adulthood. We presume we know all we need to know—our learning is complete. It's not.

Even we old dogs can learn new tricks, and we should. If you have figured out your Ultimate Purpose, chances are good you have some learning to do before you can fully live it. We want children to grow into lifelong learners, and we should demand the same from ourselves. Creating a personal environment where you devote time and energy to your own curiosity, self-awareness, and personal growth keeps your brain nimble. Life is more exciting when you are curious—when you want to know more, when you thirst for knowledge about yourself and your world. Over the years, I have seen caregivers take on all kinds of challenges and follow whims of curiosity. They have done things such as return to (and graduate from) college, learn to ride a bike or rock climb, overcome their fear of public speaking, change careers, and pursue a wide variety of other hobbies and pastimes. They report feeling energized, renewed, fresh, and inspired. In my own life, I find taking on new challenges gives me new perspective on my life. I feel more capable and more tuned in to the true depth of my own abilities.

Use the following activities as a foundation for feeding your curiosity, expanding your self-awareness, and focusing on your personal growth. Close your eyes and take a few deep breaths, then make a list of things about which you are curious. Don't edit yourself, just jot down things as they pop into your head. Come back and add to this list as you think of new things you want to know about.

_____

_____

_____

_____

_____

Pick two or three of the things from your list and research them. You can always finish this chapter later. The Internet is a good place to start, and you will want to use other sources of information as well. Invest some time and energy in learning what you want to know. Chances are the things you are most curious about relate to your personal growth and self-awareness in some way. Look for those connections and use the space provided to jot any necessary notes.

_____

_____

_____

_____

Make a point of finding answers to all the things you listed that you are curious about. You will find some of them lead to more curiosities. Follow up on those as well and see where they lead you.

Do Your Environments Allow for Both Group and Alone Time?

Socialization is important for young children, but they also need time alone to process all the information their busy brains acquire during the course of a day full of play, exploration, and discovery. They need downtime to recharge, regroup, and relax. So do you.

The problem is you probably don't have more than a few minutes to yourself on an average day. Being a caregiver means that other people usually surround you while you struggle to make sure they have all they need from life at any given moment. New parents usually have a hard time understanding that they need to spend time away from their baby now and then. They do not understand that time away allows them to recharge, decompress, and take the edge off. Most experienced caregivers know they need this kind of time to themselves as well, but many just don't take it.

I know parents who make time for regular date nights and individual alone time. I know caregivers who manage to carve out regular time for hiking, sewing, reading, music, martial arts, gardening, and a long list of other pastimes. When asked how they make the time, most have said they just make it happen. Some get up early. Others go to bed a bit late. Some organize their lives more efficiently to allow for some personal time. Others just sneak off from their lives occasionally for their alone time. The point most make is that they value the escape so much they are able to work it into their schedules. They also say escaping gets easier with practice. One family child care provider shared with me, "The first time I made time to go off for a long walk all by myself I felt terribly guilty walking out the door, but by the time I came home I was refreshed. Now it is something I just have to do because I know I am better at work and life afterwards."

Another thing many of us need is more time away from children, time when we do not think about children, talk about children, and worry about children. It is good to make time in your life for hobbies, events, and activities that have nothing to do with those snotty little curtain-climbing, crumb-dropping drool machines we love so much. I have met groups of providers who schedule regular "girls' nights" when they go out and have a meal, a few drinks, and a lot of conversation. The only rule is that the conversation cannot be about children or work. Some couples I have met report abiding by the same rule during their date nights. My own experience is that getting totally away from the job makes me better at that job when I return to it. Here are some things that might help you create more personal time in your life:

1. Learn to say "no" to the things in your life you really do not have time for. Taking on fewer projects frees up time that you can then invest in yourself. Like so many other

things, this is easy for me to suggest but not so easy to do in real life. Saying no is not simple; it can be scary. It is so hard to do in real life because in real life we have to deal with the fallout. Depending on who you are saying no to, you may experience emotions such as fear, guilt, and anxiety when contemplating a *no*. If you are known as an easy *yes* and then start saying *no* to people, they will have to make adjustments in their lives, which can lead to more fallout you have to navigate.

Here's a tip: start small, and pick an easy *no* to start with. Another tip is to practice in your own head before you do it for real. Visualizing yourself saying no and handling the fallout well will make it easier when you do it in real life. You should also trust your gut when deciding who and what to say no to. It will not be easy at first—change never is—but in the end you gain more control of your life, add some time to your schedule, and build your confidence. After she got comfortable saying *no* to things, one mother I know described it as "becoming a whole new me."

2. Block off a small amount of time for yourself in your schedule every day to read, meditate, listen to music, or just sit quietly in the sunshine.

3. Schedule weekly adult time for dinner, dancing, bike riding, walking, or a hobby. The only rule is no kids.

4. Give yourself permission to be a bit selfish. Type into your computer, write on a scrap of paper, or yell out the window, "It is okay for me to be a bit selfish and take some of *my* time for *myself*!"

Also, consider the following:

List three decadently selfish things you would like to make time for in your life.

_____

_____

_____

What major road blocks are keeping you from your decadently selfish behavior?

_____

_____

_____

What strategies can get you over, under, around, or through those road blocks?

_____

_____

_____

Do Your Environments Foster Trusting Relationships?

Children need to trust their caregivers before they really feel comfortable and able to take learning risks in a child care program. Annie and Siddha are able to go off and explore the world with such ease because they trust me to keep them safe, set limits, and assist them when needed. They are confident I will not let flower shop cats and garbage trucks hurt them, which means they are free to explore the world and learn what they need to know.

We adults need the same trusting relationships that children are so dependent on. Everything my friend Chris taught me would have been meaningless to me if I hadn't trusted him. My trust in Tasha to support me, tell me when I am being a jerk, and love me unconditionally keeps me going every day. We need to nurture such relationships, but too often we hide from them. On some level, trusting another person makes you vulnerable; it is a risk. We worry about being ridiculed, looked down on, laughed at, stabbed in the back, or marginalized. Therefore, instead of opening up and trusting, we stay closed and push people away. We build walls and moats around ourselves in an effort to seem invulnerable.

Here are some questions and writing assignments to help you understand your thinking about trusting relationships a bit better:

Who are the people in your life you trust the most and why?

_____

_____

_____

Write about a time when you were hurt or deceived by someone close to you that you trusted.

_____

_____

_____

How has that incident affected your ability to trust other people?

_____

_____

_____

What is the scariest thing about trusting new acquaintances?

_____

_____

_____

Write about the last time you let down someone who trusted you, and explain how you felt about that incident.

_____

_____

_____

List some ideas that could help you become more trusting of the people closest to you.

_____

_____

_____

_____

The whole idea of trusting yourself or other people can be scary or overwhelming. One small step you can take to become more trusting is to catch yourself second-guessing your inner voice. Most of the time that voice is a reliable assessor of your situation. Learning to trust that voice also means you will know when you are in a situation in which you really shouldn't be so trusting. You can also try to catch yourself *not* trusting. Then ask yourself why you are doing so in that situation. Understanding why you don't trust can be useful in developing new behaviors and interpersonal practices. It is also a good idea to think about people, situations, and thoughts you do trust. Then you can examine why trusting is possible at some times and not at others.

As with children's environments, adult environments—both physical and emotional—are healthier, happier, and more productive when we trust the people around us. Taking some time to understand our own history with trusting relationships can go a long way in improving our current feelings and explaining our actions. This is not easy stuff to think about; if it were, we would be thinking about it all the time. Building trust is all about balancing your personal fears and your temperament with your need to be close to other people. It takes work, but you can build more trusting relationships.

Tactics, Tools, and Tips

1. Since the beginning of this book, I have been encouraging you to take deep cleansing breaths to help clear and focus your mind, but breathing through your worry, stress, tension, frustration, and fear is not easy. Sometimes the chatter and

clutter are overwhelming and finding focus seems impossible. Here is a simple activity to help keep your mind in the moment:

- Sit comfortably and breathe normally.

- Begin counting to yourself, quietly saying the next number in your head with each exhalation.

- When you reach 25, begin counting backwards to zero.

- If your mind wanders, gently bring it back to the task and begin counting again with the number you were on before.

- To challenge yourself, count to 50, 100, or 200 and then back to zero. Another challenge is to count by 2s, 3s, or 7s.

This activity gives the mind a simple task to occupy itself and keep from roaming all over time and space. It should leave you feeling calm, relaxed, and ready to engage with your environment.

2. Reflective practice is the regular review and revision of the way we do things in order to improve how we do them. This is a key aspect of professionalism. It is also a key aspect in maintaining your smile. Develop the habit of routinely stepping back and assessing how you do what you do, and then make adjustments as needed. It is a way to ensure you are on the right track in your life, a way to determine if you are making progress toward your goals. You can do this in your head if you like, but you may want to consider using a notebook to track your thoughts, insights, and ideas about the ways you do things.

3. You are a work in progress. Living your Ultimate Purpose, changing your mind-set, and enriching your physical and emotional environments is challenging and does not happen overnight. Here are two ideas to help keep you on task and headed in the right direction:

- Set intentions: Make it a routine to spend three minutes before bed every night listing your intentions for the coming day. Your intentions could be simple tasks that move you through life or toward your Ultimate Purpose such as "I intend to get groceries," "I intend to walk the dog three miles," or "I intend to pay the phone bill." They also could be broader ideas that influence your interactions with the world, such as "I intend to be more open to other people's ideas," "I intend to really listen when Larry talks to me," or "I intend to take three deep breaths before I speak when I am upset." Look at these intentions as your wishes for the coming day. Then get a good night's sleep, and make those wishes come true.

- Run mental simulations: One hard thing about making changes is that you never know what is going to happen next when you leave your comfort zone. Running mental simulations of new activities or endeavors before taking them on in real life is a good way to prepare mentally for the unknown. It's easy—just sit comfortably and visualize yourself doing whatever needs to be done. Make the picture real by adding as much sensory detail as possible. Play this simulation in your head repeatedly until you feel confident and ready to tackle your next challenge.

4. Earlier in this chapter, I wrote about the impact clutter can have on your happiness, outlook, and progress toward your goals. The problem is that reining in the clutter in your life can seem overwhelming and beyond your powers. Here are some tips to help nudge you in the right direction:

- Break big jobs down into bite-size bits. Don't plan to spend an entire weekend organizing the whole house and then feel guilty when you don't accomplish everything you planned. Instead, break the job into small pieces and spend 20 minutes a day on those small pieces. This way the job is not as overwhelming, you have a little victory every day, and over time you see big results.

- Toss junk mail as soon as you get it instead of letting it pile up on the kitchen counter until the dog is accidently buried in an avalanche of credit card applications and pizza coupons. Do the same with your e-mail inbox—if it is junk, delete it.

- Sort items into four groups and then deal with them accordingly: garbage (not useful), recycle (useful to someone else), valuable (has physical or emotional value), don't know (things you can't make a decision about).

- Be tough on yourself. If you really want to de-clutter your space, you are going to have to make some hard choices. Is there any reason that fruitcake Aunt Bessie gave you back in 1997 is still on the kitchen counter? Are you ever going to re-read the six years worth of old newspapers in the garage? Will there ever be another hamster in your life or can you get rid of the cage? Making the tough calls might not be easy in the moment, but after the fact, you will be proud of yourself.

- Stop buying stuff. One reason we end up drowning in clutter is that we buy things we don't really need and don't have room for in our lives. Shopping fills an emotional void for many people. It is a lot easier to go to the mall than it is to deal with what is eating at us.

- Remember that doing away with clutter is hard work. It requires you to replace old habits with new habits. It takes time. You might want to consider teaming with a friend who is also trying to manage his mess. The support of someone to keep you on track is a valuable resource.

5. To get more in tune with your physical and emotional environments, get completely away from them once in a while. Escaping from your "normal" life full of habits, predictability, and comfortable routine can be refreshing. This is why vacations are so rejuvenating. They are chances to get away from regular environments, think novel thoughts, behave differently, try on new habits, and explore parts of your identity that are seldom part of your regular life.

   I realize that you probably can't jet off to the south of France this weekend or run away to the green sandy beach of an exotic island for a month, but you can get away from it all for a while. You don't have to do something big, just do something different—shake things up, climb outside your box, try something new, explore your possibilities, act out of character. I don't know what "different" looks like to you, so I can't make any specific suggestions about what you should do. I just know that spending time away from your normal life in a fresh and stimulating environment will do you worlds of good. It will not only open your eyes to new possibilities, it will help you appreciate the good parts of your regular life. Your assignment? Make and implement plans to shake things up a little bit. Have some fun.

Seven
Building
Your Balance

SOMETIMES I WISH I HAD one of those perfect lives it looks like other people are living—a life where every day is flawless from dawn until dusk, a life in which nothing irritates me, nothing goes wrong, nothing stresses me, nothing raises my blood pressure, nothing scratches at my last nerve, nothing eats at me, and nothing weighs me down. In my perfect life

- there aren't always bills in the mail;
- traffic lights are always in sync and always green;
- the neighbor's big dog does not poop big poops in my yard;
- I look like George Clooney and have Donald Trump's money;
- I always know what to say and how to act;
- the weather is always the weather I want;
- I don't have to take my shoes off at the airport;
- chocolate cake is healthy;
- my life is filled with exactly what I want when I want it.

I'm sure it does not come as a shock to hear that I do not have that life. No one does. Not even the people who look like they are living perfect lives have perfect lives. Even Mr. George Clooney with his looks, fame, and fortune has to deal with the paparazzi constantly following him around taking his picture, making his very public life even more public.

What we all need more of in our lives is balance. If you don't believe me, look at these synonyms for the word balance and think about whether you want more of these things in your life, or not:

- equilibrium
- poise
- stability
- steadiness
- symmetry
- evenness
- harmony

These things are what most of us are searching for—the things that make us smile. Lack of these things leads to stress, frustration, resentment, hurt, anger, and all those other feelings that eat away at us. If you want lasting happiness, you have to make adjustments to improve your balance. *Improving* your balance should be your goal, because perfecting it is impossible. No matter how hard you try, you cannot reach perfection. Life always tosses you an unexpected challenge now and then that makes you wobble. Kids are going to puke on your shoes, tires are going to go flat on dark and stormy nights, relationships are going to form or fall apart, and every once in a while a seagull is going to poop on your head as you enjoy a day at the beach. Life happens, and sometimes it is a pain in the butt. This is why it is important to have healthy habits and effective practices you can rely on when the going gets tough. As you commit to caring for yourself, you learn to bounce back from life's surprises quicker and more efficiently. You are destined to spend the rest of your life seeking equilibrium and adjusting your balance.

Can Good Enough Be Good Enough?

Better balance can make your life happier, but it can never make it perfect. One of the first adjustments we need to make has to do with our view of perfection. Wanting things to be perfect is one thing. I am all for striving for perfection and wanting the best, but expectations of perfection can make our balance falter, because true perfection is unachievable. I have met many caregivers who have set unattainably high expectations for themselves and the people around them. They need to be perfect, the children in their care need to be perfect, their sweetie needs to be perfect, their dog needs to be perfect, but try as they might, no one is ever perfect enough. The fact that no one ever manages to live up to these high expectations causes a lot of discord and stress.

Here are some questions to consider:

Think for a moment about the standards you set for yourself and others. How do those standards affect your personal actions and interactions?

Where did the standards you have for yourself and others come from?

How do those tendencies affect your relationships?

In which areas of your life could you lower your standards and be happy with what is good enough? What would "good enough" look like? How will you know when you have reached it in each area?

BALANCE-O-MATIC

Life gets busy, leaving us feeling flustered and out of balance. Make way for the Balance-O-Matic. With a simple, same-day surgery to implant microscopic emotional gyroscopes in each of your inner ears and a microprocessor relay on the surface of your cerebral cortex, we can effectively create an emotional early warning system that signals you when your life slips out of balance. The deluxe package also includes the implantation of a neural shock system that delivers a small electrical jolt—literally shocking you into caring for yourself—if you fail to take balance-restoring action in a reasonable amount of time.

The Balance-O-Matic helps restore a healthy balance between your work life and nonwork life—reducing stress, relieving anxiety, and realigning focus. Buy yours today!

Are You a Crawdad?

At a conference in Kansas a few years ago a child care provider said she "tried not to be a crawdad" as a strategy for keeping her smile. My experience with crawdads is limited to watching Granny fix a batch of them on *The Beverly Hillbillies,* so I did not immediately grasp the point she was making. She explained that when she was a kid she and her friends would go to a nearby stream or pond and coax crawdads, which look like minilobsters, to grab hold of sticks. They would dangle the sticks in front of the little critters until they grabbed hold. The neat thing was that the feisty crustaceans would not willingly let go. They held tight to the stick for a long time, assuming it was food and not wanting it to escape. She didn't want to be a crawdad, so she made a point of letting go of things in her life she did not need to hold onto any longer. This brought more balance to her life than holding on.

A desire not to be a crawdad—a willingness to let go—would do a lot of us good. We tend to hold onto all kinds of things and allow them to weigh us down. There are ideas, thoughts, people, and feelings we should let go of after a while. We hold onto lots of things way too long, and it affects our balance. I wrote in a previous chapter about how I took on a lot of projects after my dad's death as a way of avoiding the hurt I was feeling. Instead of dealing with the hurt, I ignored it. This threw me out of balance for some time, and things only got better after I acknowledged the hurt. That acknowledgement was the first little step toward bringing my balance back. Then I was gradually able to work through the grieving process, letting go of my hurt, anger, disappointment, self-blame, and all the rest.

Knowing what to let go of or add more of to bring about balance in your life is not always easy, mainly because it is so difficult to see when you are out of balance. Listening to that little voice inside your head—trusting your intuition—is a first step. When you listen closely, you get a feeling for what you need more of or less of in your life. You also get an idea of the changes you need to make to gain more balance. Take a look at your crawdadness:

List three types of things you tend to hold onto for too long.

_____

_____

_____

Why do you hold onto these things?

_____

_____

_____

How does holding onto these things affect balance in your life?

_____

_____

_____

_____

What would make it easier for you to let go of these things?

_____

_____

_____

_____

Where Are You Looking?

Balance would be easy if there was some sort of calculation you could perform or multiple-choice test you could take to determine if you had it, but that is not the case. Balance is hard to quantify—my balance might not be your balance. Balance is unique to the individual, like a fingerprint, neural map, or retinal scan. Our fingertips, brains, and eyes might be similar, but they are also very different. So are our ideas of balance.

You can't test for it, but you can feel it. If you spend some time looking inside your head, listening to the things rattling around in there and paying close attention, you will begin to feel where you are in and out of balance. You have an inner awareness that is always trying to convey this information. The problem is you are not always listening. The clutter and chaos of everyday life sometimes make tuning in to your awareness difficult. It's hard to devote much time during the day to listening to your inner voice when you're responsible for the well-being and safety of half a dozen curious, energetic, and loud toddlers. The outer world demands so much attention that we don't give our inner worlds their due. We do not devote enough attention to what our minds are trying to tell us. Feelings about balance are there; we are just missing the messages.

Take a few moments right now and let your eyes rest. Breathe deeply. Clear your head. Listen to your inner awareness. It might come quickly, or it might take some time. But you will connect with a clear feeling about how balanced your life is right now in this moment. Pay close attention. As you tune to that feeling, you may realize some areas of life are more unbalanced than other areas. Maybe work is fine, but home is chaos. Maybe you realize you are not paying enough attention to a particular person or responsibility. Maybe you realize you are hiding from a problem that needs addressing. Maybe you feel life is closing in on you.

It may be hard, but stick with these feelings. Continue to look inward. Continue to seek the things in your life that really matter, and determine if they are getting enough of your attention. Continue this self-inquiry a bit longer—until you feel you have gained a superior understanding of the state of your personal emotional equilibrium, then slowly open your eyes and take a few minutes to jot down any insights you may have gained.

I know a parent—I'll call her Molly—who described her life as *claustrophobic*. She loved her three children, but as a single mom, she felt like sometimes the only things she ever did were work and parent. This feeling led to lots of guilt. She felt like a bad mommy for now and then wanting to be away from her children and her role as a parent. After she shared this feeling, I encouraged her to just spend some time sitting and feeling it, not hiding from it or overworking herself in an attempt to escape it.

She gave it a try. Over time, she realized she was somebody more than a mother and an employee. She was a unique and special person, not just a prop in the lives of others. I have to stress that it was not easy for her—it took effort and time—but it did lead to positive changes in her life. Molly eventually started setting aside time for her needs, dreams, and desires. She let go of her guilt. She invested in her own happiness. She realized her efforts made her "a happier mother" and she felt "more tuned in" to the needs of her children. She had thought taking care of herself was a selfish act, but it turned out not only that it made her a happier individual but a better parent.

It is my hope that you can get a feel for when your balance is good and when it needs attention. Looking inward is the only real way to figure this out. There is no way *I* can tell *you* what parts of *your* life want more balance. Looking inward and finding balance in your life should feel empowering, because at its core it is a way for you to take control of your life. It is a way for you to see what areas of your life need attention and what kind of attention is needed. Then you can move yourself toward some sort of positive action. Lack of this kind of control over your life may be one of the core things you feel you have been missing. Too often we feel like life is happening to us and we are without any means to control events. Tuning into your feelings about balance is an easy process that can be very empowering if you are open to the experience. It might take some practice, but you are worth the investment of time involved.

Molly didn't do it overnight. It took a great deal of self searching and thought about her life, and it led her to a better place. She went from watching her life as an outsider—reacting to events as they unfolded and feeling little or no control—to actively living her life with a newborn sense of purpose.

You may want to consider the mind of a toddler. You know how very adept they are at seeing useful knowledge and skills and then integrating them into their lives. They are always assessing their surroundings and taking personally beneficial actions. I'm amazed at how quickly their busy brains assimilate knowledge. They are wired to pick up language, ideas, and helpful knowledge about how to operate effectively in the world in which they live. Just look at the changes in language skills, physical skills, and knowledge of their surroundings a child goes through between the ages of one and two-and-a-half. It is my hope that you can be as attuned to your needs and able to meet those needs as an average toddler.

Where Is Your Attention?

As I mentioned earlier, if you can invest time in taking care of your hair and teeth every day, you should be able to find five or ten minutes to invest in taking care of yourself emotionally. This is often difficult because we are so busy focusing on immediate demands for our attention that we are unable to find time to focus on our long-term welfare. Thinking about your personal emotional needs is difficult when cute little Sally is across the room trying to pick up the hamster with a vacuum cleaner while her brother Vinnie is sticking self-adhesive googly eyes to his butt.

When you work to get a feel for your balance, you may find that your attention needs your attention. You may find you are always living moment to moment, putting out one fire after another, handling one emergency and then zipping to the next. You may find you are always saving hamsters and prying self-adhesive googly eyes off little butts. You may find you are living most of your day with hurried immediacy.

I believe we need to learn to live in the moment. We need to tune in to the here and now. We need to quit worrying about the past and fretting about the future and be present in the present. Sometimes, however, learning to get away from *right now* once in a while is a good thing. Living from emergency to emergency is overwhelming. Make time to step back from the chaos and pay attention to your short- and long-term needs. Think about what you need from your life over the next few days, weeks, and years. Look at the big picture of your life. Step back from the roadblocks you are always encountering and plan ways around, over, under, or through them.

Right now I would like you to commit to spending some time thinking about what you need in your life. In the next forty-eight hours, I want you to get away from the chaos of your life in some way. You can go for a walk, take a bubble bath, sit in a dark room listening to your iPod, or take a drive down a quiet country road. The goal is to get into your own head. After thirty minutes or so into this activity, I want you to make a list of what you need in the next week, the next 30 days, and the next year. Then I want you to keep your list handy and refer to it frequently. Use it as a guide when you feel like you are drifting and need to center your thinking.

Getting out of the moment and seeing the big picture may actually lead to fewer fires when you go back to living in the moment. You may see strategies and tactics to solve some of the problems you are always confronting that you could not see when you were so close to those problems. Maybe the hamster and the vacuum should not be accessible at the same time. Maybe you need to buy glue-on googly eyes instead of the self-adhesive ones.

The point is, sometimes we find balance by taking our attention out of the moment and focusing on the bigger picture. Getting away from the immediacy of *right now* is something lots of caregivers need, especially when working with highly demanding young children.

I spent nearly one-third of the first quarter of 2009 in hotels. Easter weekend 2009 was my first weekend at home in over two months. I'd been traveling a lot talking to child care providers and parents about early learning and about investing time in their own care and well-being. I'd met many inspiring, energetic, passionate, and dedicated expert caregivers over the last few months, and they invigorated me professionally. I love speaking and enjoy the travel, but I have to admit I was really looking forward to a three-day weekend at home, a chance to spend some time away from other people's children and away from writing, speaking, and traveling.

It was wonderful. I started renovating my woodworking shop, which meant ripping out walls and making five trips to the dump to dispose of the debris. It was hard work, but it was fun. I also had time to go for a long bike ride, covering 20 miles of local bike paths on a beautiful spring day. Feeling the warm sun on my skin as I pedaled along was exhilarating. On Easter Sunday I got to encourage my nieces to sneak candy when their mom was not looking, let them play with our pet turtle, and allow them to run in the house; I did everything I could to rile them up before sending them home. I love working with kids, but I have to admit they can be a lot more entertaining after I've had a glass of good wine. It was fun to ignore some of the rules, regulations, and expectations we have in our child care program, to be a bit more wild and goofy and to not be a professional role model for a little while.

I also went on a date with Tasha to the post office to apply for passports. It was not a fancy date, but it was fun to spend time together on something not related to children or child care. I invited her to go to the dump with me a couple of times, but she declined. I guess the idea of two dates in one weekend was just more than she could handle.

In addition to all this, I found some time to read, ignored my e-mail and computer, and did some writing. As you can see, I am not only a really romantic guy, I am also a really boring guy. Most of my first weekend to myself in months was spent running errands, working in my garage, and pedaling around on my bike. I am not a wild and crazy guy by a long shot.

So what's the point of sharing a boring sketch of my much needed but mildly mundane weekend at home? The point is that

I loved and savored every second of it. It felt good. It was refreshing, invigorating, and enjoyable. It recharged me physically and mentally. The intense physicality of the demolition and bike riding is something I don't get enough of as a family child care provider, speaker, and author. Just being an uncle instead of an early care and education professional was also a pleasant change from my usual routine.

Now, I have to ask: When was the last time you took a three-day weekend for yourself? When was the last time you made time to engage in activities you enjoy? When was the last time you took off your early care and education professional hat for a few days? When was the last time you devoted an extended hunk of time to doing something for yourself?

If it has been awhile, I have to tell you, you need to try it. I make a bit of time for myself every day, and I work hard to ensure I manage my stress well. But that big glob of unscheduled free time I got Easter weekend was special, and you should try it out if you haven't done so for a long time.

I know the excuses: "I don't have time." "I feel selfish taking time for myself." "There is so much work to do." "There is a grant proposal due on Monday." "I feel guilty." I also know that often you need permission to take care of yourself.

Well, take a deep breath and forget about all those things. Be a little selfish, let go of the guilt, and push the paperwork aside. If you need permission to take care of yourself, I hereby grant it. Get out your calendar right now, and schedule some time for yourself.

Is It a Need or a Want?

Some children have a hard time distinguishing between the letters *p, b,* and *d,* and some adults have the same problem with wants and needs. This confusion of wants and needs is the cause for some people's imbalance. Sometimes we mistakenly think we need things that are really wants—flat screen TVs, fancy cars, iPhones, and other people's approval. I believe life is more balanced when we are able to draw a distinct line between what we need and what we want:

1. I *need* a reliable way to get from point A to point B, but I *want* a yellow convertible.
2. I *need* to take some time off from work so I can stay balanced, but I *want* to go to Hawaii for three weeks.
3. I *need* to eat something, but I *want* a half gallon of homemade chocolate ice cream.

For the sake of clarity, let's define a *need* as something necessary for physical and emotional survival and a *want* as something that is desired. The balance I have established in my life ends if I am consumed by my desire for a flashy car, a long beach vacation, and too much ice cream. Giving in to those wants would lead me to speeding tickets, debt, and bigger pants. Letting wants masquerade as needs gives them more power over our lives than they deserve. It is important to clarify which is which if we want to live in balance. I may have that car and take that vacation someday, but I am not going to let my desire for them consume me or draw my attention away from my real needs.

Use the space provided to clarify your own needs and wants:

To lead a happy life, I *need* . . .

_____

_____

To lead a happy life, I *want* . . .

_____

_____

Add or subtract items from these lists as time goes by, and refer to them often. They may come in handy when you are struggling with certain decisions about how to spend your time, energy, and other resources.

Can You Find the Space You Need?

Does life, at times, leave you feeling claustrophobic? Do you feel like the walls are closing in, like you are drowning, or like the physical and emotional space you *have* is not the space you *need*? On a visit to the east coast, I met an assistant teacher in a pre-school classroom who described feeling "submerged" in her job and said she had moments when she felt as if she were "suffocating, breathing in the same old stale air day after day." I've met some young stay-at-home moms who described similar feelings. One talked about how she was "chained to the house and baby," and another said she needed "to see what was on the other side of the fence" she had built around her little family. A third mommy, with a beautiful two-year-old son and a newborn daughter, said her head was "so cluttered that I can't find space to move in there."

The clutter of our mental space and the confining feelings we get from our physical space can cause a lot of mental turbulence. Feeling these things consistently can really throw our balance off. Sometime we need to abandon the confines we feel trapped in and seek wide-open spaces. In elementary school, I used to get in trouble a lot for daydreaming. I would tune out what was happening in the classroom and escape into my head or out the window. Both escape routes offered broad, spacious freedom from mundane worksheets and the smell of chalk dust.

If you are feeling confined in your head or your physical space, I encourage you to find better balance by seeking wide-open spaces. Quit isolating yourself; become of the world. If you have habitually closed yourself off from the world, it takes some effort to be part of it again, but doing so is very empowering. We need to spend time in our nests, and we also need to fly. Here are some things to think about:

Do you feel you are always either at home or at work? If so, where else could you go to break that cycle?

_____

_____

_____

_____

_____

What three activities would make your physical and mental life feel more spacious?

_____

_____

_____

What are four things that make you feel most emotionally confined?

_____

_____

_____

Would there be anything wrong with putting this book down right now and going for a short walk or connecting with a friend you have not spoken to in a while? If you can't do it, why not? If you can, why are you still reading?

_____

_____

_____

Are You Always Carrying a Bag?

Sometimes we get out of balance because of the baggage we carry from place to place. We bring home to work and work to home. We lug that argument we had with coworkers or family around for weeks, months, and even years. We haul around the expectations others have for us. We tote our personal shortcomings and perceived failures. Some of this is big stuff concerning death, abuse, heartbreak, bad choices, and loss. But much of it is trivial. Sometimes I still feel a bit ticked off at a girl from elementary school—though I can't even remember her name—who used to tease me about my pointy ears and big nose.

What's more, we often end up carrying other people's baggage too. One reason so many of us are caregivers is we are innately empathetic. We are good at tuning in to other people's emotions, at connecting to their feelings. This means people open up to us and share things they might not share with others. I know too much about some people I don't know too well, and it weighs on me sometimes. When others share, we end up feeling their emotions. This comes in handy when tuning in to a child, but it is not a good thing when we end up sharing the emotional lives of too many people.

I frequently hear from caregivers about how parents share way too much information. "They trust me with their children, and I guess that means they feel comfortable trusting me with their secrets and problems too," one provider said. She had recently dealt with a situation in which the mother of a two-year-old in her child care confided she was having an affair with her boss. The mother wanted this caregiver to cover for her if her husband started asking questions. The caregiver refused to take part in the subterfuge, but she had a hard time letting go of the disappointment and anger she felt toward the mother. She carried around the emotional baggage for weeks. She used prayer to help put down the bundle of emotions she was hauling. Others use exercise, meditation, hobbies, or other practices to put down their heavy loads. It is not easy, and what works for one person may not work for another. You have to find your own ways of putting down your burdens. Then you have to practice. Practice will not make you perfect (there still may be things you cannot put down), but it will make you capable of releasing some of the burdens life places on your shoulders.

Our own lives are easier to balance when we can put down some of the baggage we are hauling. Think about putting down some of your load. Consider the following questions:

What are your three heaviest emotional loads right now, and how long have you been carrying each of them?

What are the biggest loads you are carrying for others, and how long have they been weighing you down?

_____

_____

_____

Which of these loads can you safely put down?

_____

Who could you trust to help with your load?

_____

How can you approach them for help?

_____

Do You Get Physical?

While many of us get some exercise chasing children around all day long, we probably do not get as much as we need to live long, healthy lives. After a long, hard day with children, it is too easy to flip on the television, grab a bag of chips, and spend four or five hours watching _Law & Order_ reruns. When we get time to ourselves, we like to veg out. Passively watching television and munching chips from time to time is not bad, but it can easily become a habit that knocks your body out of balance.

I would like you to consider getting a bit more physical in your free time. Go for a walk, do some gardening, take a bike ride, go dancing, jump rope, or use a hula hoop. Physical activity is good for your heart, lungs, and brain. Getting more of it makes you healthier and happier. If you are fairly active and get plenty of exercise, make sure you hold on for the long term to the activities you engage in. When life gets hectic and hard it is very easy to let healthy habits slip away.

Use the space provided to list three or four physical activities you enjoy but have not made enough time for recently. Then put this book down and go do one of those activities. Make the activity more fun by inviting your sweetie or a friend to join you. This shared time will be good for your relationship, which is something I address in the next chapter.

_____

_____

_____

_____

_____

Need a *Special Moment*?

Speaking of getting physical, my wife, Tasha, and I have conducted extensive research into sex since 1986. In that time, we have reached some definitive conclusions:

- Practice *does* make perfect.
- Sex with the same person over and over again only gets boring if you let it get boring.
- Sex can lead to children and children can get in the way of sex.
- Sex can help you sleep, clear your sinuses, and relieve headaches.
- There is a clear link between sex and stress.

While I feel confident enough to write in detail on all of these research results, I am going to focus my attention on the last one, the link between sex and stress. Sometimes sex is the cause of stress, and sometimes sex is a great stress reliever.

There have been times in my relationship with Tasha when we have let stress from life seep between the sheets. Carrying the weight of the world into the bedroom is a great way to kill the mood. The fact that I spent many years expecting Tasha to be frisky and ready to go whenever I was in the mood didn't help the situation. Let's state the obvious: guys and gals look at sex differently. Over the years, I've learned from Tasha that even the idea of sex could be stressful:

- Sometimes she just feels fat and unsexy.

- Sometimes sex seems like just another chore on a long to-do list, just one more thing that needs doing.

- Sometimes the prep work—shaving, fixing her hair, putting on lotion and perfume, applying lipstick, doing her nails, finding something sexy to wear that (as Tasha says) makes her "boobs and butt look good"—is more work than it is worth.

- Sometimes not being an eighteen-year-old—or not having a body that looks and works like it did when it was eighteen—makes her sad.

- Sometimes being quiet is hard. When the kids were little, Tasha did not want to wake them, and now that they are older, she does not want them to know (hear) what is going on.

If you are stressed out to start with and feel sex is another chore with its own set of stressors, getting in the mood is difficult. On the other hand, climbing between the sheets and having a *special moment* with your sweetie is a good way to let go of the weight of the world. It's hard to think about toast crumbs and dirty dishes on the kitchen counter when your back is arching and your toes are curling during a *special moment*. Science has shown that sex releases happy chemicals in the brain, gets the heart pumping, renews your connection with your sweetie, and clears the mind. A fulfilling sex life with someone you love is a great way to keep your smile.

Your sex life, like the rest of your life, needs balance. Here are some tips to help you find that balance:

- Make time for *special moments*: It might not seem romantic, but if you have to sit down with your sweetie and schedule some intimate physical time then do it. Pick a time, date, and location and mark it on your calendar with a big smiley face. Anticipating such a get-together may have both of you smiling all day long.

- Break your routine: Find ways to keep your relationship fresh and new. Do whatever it takes to shake things up a bit and add some excitement to your relationship.

- Flirt: This works best when you flirt with *your* sweetie. We too often let our relationships get stagnate. We take them for granted and become stuck in routines. Fight this by spicing things up. Consider making eyes at each other, leaving each other love notes, or surprising each other with little gifts. After over twenty years together, Tasha can look at me in a way that raises my temperature, speeds my heart rate, and makes me feel twenty years younger. If you're uncomfortable with this kind of thing, I have one word of advice: practice.

- Pull your weight outside the bedroom: Doing your part to make your relationship work outside the bedroom directly affects how the relationship works between the sheets. This comes up sometimes in training sessions about stress and burnout, and it appears to me that some men would get a lot more sex if they put down the toilet seat, picked up their dirty clothes, and listened with a tad more consistency.

Now put down this silly book, go grab your sweetie by the hand, apologize for anything you need to apologize for, and then make time to share a *special moment* or two.

Tactics, Tools, and Tips

1. Bad choices often result in a loss of balance. I learned this the hard way when I was about eleven and climbed on the roof of the neighbor's garage. Gravity is a harsh mistress. When confronted with choices, asking yourself two questions can help maintain your balance. First, ask yourself, "What's the cost?" Consider how much of your time, energy, and other resources each possible choice would require. Making a realistic assessment of costs may help you make a more balanced decision.

    The second question to ask yourself is, "Will this choice bring balance or cause stress?" Balance is important for happiness, but most of the time most of us don't even consider it when making day-to-day life choices. Investing a few moments in thought can save you from hours, days, weeks, or even years of regret. Taking the time to ask these simple, thoughtful questions can make life easier. It is okay to say *no* to things that are going to disrupt the balance of your life.

2. Understanding just what it is in your life that is out of balance is not always easy. To help get a better grasp on what is messing up your balance, fill in the blanks in the following sentences. I've conveniently left three blanks for each sentence just in case you have more than one answer.

My life needs more . . .

_____

_____

_____

My life needs less . . .

_____

_____

_____

I need to begin . . .

_____

_____

_____

I need to stop . . .

_____

_____

_____

I need to continue . . .

_____

_____

_____

I need a different approach when dealing with . . .

_____

_____

_____

Review your responses to these questions and see what you have learned about how to bring equilibrium to your life.

3. Sometimes we can find more balance in our lives by re-thinking our standards a bit. When we set expectations for people, places, and things at wholly unrealistic levels, our stress levels go up and our balance goes out of whack. Sometimes the standards we set are too high and sometimes they are too low. Expecting a three-month-old puppy to be 100 percent housebroken is expecting too much. Allowing a three-year-old child to get by without picking up her toys is not expecting enough. Lowering the standards for the puppy and raising the standards for the child can both result in a more balanced life for the adult caring for them.

I spent years encouraging, begging, demanding, ordering, and scolding kids to keep the sand in the sandbox. It caused me stress, and after reevaluating my expectations, I decided that keeping the sand in the sandbox hindered play and learning. I changed my standards. Now we try to keep the sand in the yard. The result is that play is not interrupted by my scolding anymore. Everyone is more relaxed. I don't feel like a bad guy. Life is better.

Take some time to think about the standards you have set for yourself and the important people in your life. Taking a few of those long deep breaths might be a good idea right about now, as it helps clarify your thinking. Once you've thought about it, use the space provided to write about three situations in which some adjustment in your standards could lead to more balance in your life.

_____

_____

_____

_____

_____

4. What could you live without? What objects, people, activities, and ideas could you prune from your life? Use the
   space provided to make a list of these things. Often our balance is off because we are constantly tripping over things
   that are in our way. Knowing what you could do without
   is the first step in removing it from your life. Less clutter
   equals more balance.

I could live without . . .

_____

_____

_____

_____

_____

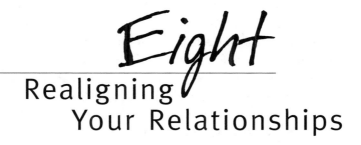Eight
Realigning
Your Relationships

MY DAUGHTER ZOË HAS BEEN a bright star in my life since her mommy and I made her back in 1993. She has put countless smiles on my face, partly because I see so much of myself in her. I have watched her grow from this perfect little baby into a smart, energetic, self-actualizing, curious, loving, funny, beautiful young woman. When she was little, she wore cute little sundresses. When we walked together, she would grab my index finger and giggle, saying "spin me daddy," as she zipped around on her toes, her dress billowing out in a colorful swirl. It has not been easy seeing her grow up. She will always be my baby, but she is no longer a baby. I have to work constantly to realign our relationship as she grows. Sometimes she reminds me, "Dad, I'm not three years old anymore!"

She is growing up, and she is outgrowing her mom and me. She doesn't need us to do all the things we have done for her over the years. Her life is getting bigger than us. She is plotting her own course in the world. Seeing her do this excites me because it is so new and fresh. I like seeing her step out into the world. On the other hand, as her daddy, I want to protect her from all the things out there that I know could hurt her. I have to hold on and let go at the same time. Time passes and relationships change. All we can do is try our best to roll with those changes.

As I've been thinking about this chapter for the last few days, another change has occurred that I am going to need to roll with.

The other day she brought The Boy home. It happened while I was at the lumberyard. Tasha told me about it, and I have to admit my heart stopped for a second—okay, two seconds.

I have known that someday The Boy would come along, and I have been preparing myself. Until he did, I hadn't fully understood the look I used to get from the fathers of girls who brought me home. It is a look of disdain, fear, hope, and surrender. The Boy sounded like a nice kid, and Zoë had been smiling for days. She repeatedly warned me to "be nice" before I met him.

The Boy walked in, looked me in the eye, and shook my hand.

"Do you smoke?" I asked.

"No."

"Do you drink?"

"No."

"Do you use drugs?"

"No."

"Do you have any kids?"

"No."

"I have two . . . and you better not hurt this one."

"Yes, sir."

"One more question. What kind of stake should I use?"

"What?"

"Well, ever since Zoë was three, I have been telling her that I was going to put the head of the first guy she brought home on a stake in the front yard as a warning to other boys. You're the first, but since I like you, I am going to let you pick what kind of stake you want me to use—oak, maple, cherry, walnut, your choice."

"I guess I'll go with a cherrywood stake."

I didn't want to like The Boy, but he seemed okay. I decided not to decapitate him right then and there, but I am keeping an eye on him.

We are responsible for the maintenance and upkeep of our own smiles, but we do not exist in a vacuum. We interact with other people all day long—our sweeties, our children, other people's children, the parents of those children, strangers, and strange boys that come sniffing around our angelic daughters. There is no way around it; we have to deal with all these people and manage the emotions they bring into our lives. These relationships can bring smiles to our faces or zap those smiles away quick as prunes through a ten-month-old.

Luckily, most of us are good at tuning in to the minds and emotions of other people. It is a skill we start developing at birth, or maybe before. Reading faces, body language, and tone of voice tells us a lot about people. I can read Tasha's mood pretty accurately by the sound of her footsteps. When she is happy she floats across a room. When she is upset or stressed her feet fall heavily like a short-circuiting robot Sasquatch walking down cast-iron stairs. We have all had lifetimes of practice reading other people, but that does not make it easy.

Keeping our relationships tuned up and properly aligned is an ongoing process and requires lots of energy. If I am tired, stressed, or out of sync, it is very difficult for me to get a good read on Tasha, even if she is stomping through the house in frustration. If we don't work at our relationships they get out of alignment and start shaking and shimmying. They begin pulling to the left or right. Steering them becomes difficult. Sometimes it feels like you're driving a sports car along a beautiful stretch of highway at sunset, and other times it feels like you're shaking along in a dilapidated old pickup toward a cliff you can't steer away from.

MANSLATOR

The Manslator is a simple device. It looks like a standard digital music player, but it's not! It records, processes, and translates all the monosyllabic grunts of man-speak into complete sentences using the poly-syllabic language women love. Just listen, and you'll be convinced!

"Humph!" becomes "Honey, I love you, but it's been a long day and I don't really want to talk about my inner feelings. All I want to do is sit in front of the flat screen and decompress."

It translates "Beer?" into "I know you're busy, and I hate to impose, but if you happen to walk by the refrigerator, please bring me a beer, some chips, and maybe some of those wonderful cookies you made last night."

"Want some?" transforms into "You're beautiful this evening! You're just as sexy as the day I met you. I love you so much even though I'm not so good at saying it sometimes. Let's make hot, wild, passionate love as soon as Tiger sinks this putt."

That's right. The Manslator turns his meaningless monosyllabic grunts and groans about TV, food, and sex into deep and meaningful utterances about TV, food, and sex. The Manslator is currently being field-tested in communities across the country and is scheduled for release next year.

Can You Rank Your Relationships?

Not all relationships are created equally. Some have a huge impact on our daily lives and require lots of resources, and others are not as demanding and have less of an impact. To better understand how your relationships have an impact on your smile, we are going to divide them into primary, secondary, and tertiary groups.

PRIMARY RELATIONSHIPS

Primary means most important, key, crucial, or main. You can have one primary relationship; one person can be most important to you. Your primary relationship is at the very top of your relationship pyramid. For most of us, our primary relationship is with our sweetie or a close adult. If you try to maintain more than one primary relationship you are probably going to have trouble somewhere along the line—ask any man with a wife and a girlfriend. Then ask the wife and the girlfriend. You'll find in most cases that trying to maintain more than one healthy primary relationship leads to stress, anger, disappointment, frustration, fear, and all kinds of messy emotions that leave you feeling tired and dirty.

Trying to maintain more than one primary relationship causes problems for a lot of couples when the stork strides through the front door with their first bouncing bundle of joy. This third party, all cute and needy and new, comes between the happy couple. One parent (usually mommy) focuses abundant time, energy, and resources on the newborn and the other parent (usually daddy) loses out. The mommy-daddy relationship suffers. New mommies and daddies are often advised to pay attention to their relationship—to make it primary—and schedule time to maintain it during those first few years of parenting. Keeping their relationship strong leads to better communication, less stress, and a healthier environment for the child.

Your primary relationship requires the most attention. Making it work takes the most effort, but it should also be the most rewarding.

SECONDARY RELATIONSHIPS

Our secondary relationships are the ones we pay a lot of attention to. These relationships include folks such as

- our own children, parents, and siblings;
- the children and parents we work with;
- friends, neighbors, peers, and coworkers.

The amount of time, energy, and resources these relationships take varies. Sometimes they are low maintenance, other times they require more work than our primary relationships. Keeping these relationships healthy is work, and it's not usually easy. The people in this group tend to compete for our attention and focus. These relationships are often very dynamic, and there can be a lot of emotional interplay among people in this group. If we are going to mess up our primary relationship, it will probably happen with someone from this group. At a recent training event, I met a young woman who was having problems because she felt her relationship with her new husband was primary and her new husband felt his relationship with his mother was primary. This young woman was very stressed out because she was forced to compete for his attention and affection.

TERTIARY RELATIONSHIPS

These relationships are the ones that form the base of our relationship pyramids. They are the relationships we have with all the people we interact with but are not especially close to, like the clerk at the grocery store, the barista at the coffee shop, other drivers on the expressway, friends of friends, and the old guy you nod a greeting to when you are out for your morning walk. These relationships are low maintenance and require few resources.

Here are some questions to ask yourself about your relationships:

Who is your one primary relationship with? Why?

_____

_____

Did you have trouble picking one name to list above? If so, who else was vying for that position and why?

_____

_____

What is the hardest thing about maintaining your primary relationship and why?

_____

_____

_____

What one thing could you do today to nurture that relationship?

_____

_____

_____

Who is your most stable secondary relationship with? What makes that relationship work? What can you learn from that relationship to strengthen other relationships?

_____

_____

_____

How Is Your Relationship with *You*?

If your relationships with others can be represented as a pyramid, your relationship with yourself should be looked at as a sphere surrounding that pyramid. Your relationship with yourself engulfs all your other relationships. If you are unhappy, insecure, befuddled, stressed, or empty, it affects every interaction you have with every person you relate to. The first step in making your relationships work is getting comfortable with yourself. The more secure you are as an individual, the healthier your relationships. That is why so much of this book has been devoted to introspection, finding balance, and knowing your Ultimate Purpose. These things all play a part in how we interact with the world.

When you are feeling bad, you're less able to know your own mind, more likely to overreact, unable to pick up on and translate other people's body language, and disadvantaged when it comes to tuning in to the minds of others. Your fear, stress, or whatever-it-is that has taken your smile acts like a thick cloud, concealing useful information you would quickly pick up on if your mind was clear and at peace. If you come home in a bad mood and your sweetie comes home in a bad mood, it is difficult for the two of you to communicate effectively. When this happens over and over, it tends to tear at the relationship. Putting your head in the right place, however, gives you a chance to defuse or avoid tough interpersonal situations because you have more information and can use it more effectively.

The most important thing that you can do to maintain, repair, and grow relationships is to care for yourself physically and emotionally. This may seem selfish, but you need to look at self-care as an investment in your relationships. The twenty to thirty minutes I spend doing yoga and meditation each morning has a direct, positive impact on every interaction I have throughout the day. Being comfortable in your own skin allows you to be more open, responsive, thoughtful, intuitive, receptive, focused, and positive. You cannot underestimate the importance of taking care of yourself when navigating your relationships. Being happy with yourself means being happier with everyone around you.

Toast or Warm Bread?

Then again, taking care of yourself sounds like a lot of work. Maybe you are thinking that it would be easier to fix all the people around you. If you can fix all the things that are wrong with other people then you won't have to deal with all the things that are wrong with you. If you could just make Bart Simpson talk more politely, get B. A. Baracus to deal with his anger and fear of flying, convince MacGyver to stop blowing things up, teach those Duke boys to obey the traffic laws, educate the Skipper about healthy eating habits and controlling his temper, and fix Monk's OCD, life will be just fine. Except it won't. You cannot fix other people. Even if you could, you would not have time to fix everything you think is wrong with everyone around you. If you spend time thinking about all the things that bug you about other people—all the things you would fix if you could—you will blow a fuse. The world is full of really messed up, irritating, irksome people.

You can't change them, but you can change the way you react to and interact with them. Here is an example from my own life. Tasha doesn't like toast, but she does like to use the toaster to make warm bread. She calls it toast, but I adamantly disagree. For it to be toast, I think in addition to the change in the bread's temperature there has to be some change in the color and texture of the bread. There has to be some *toasting*; otherwise, it is not toast, it is just warm bread. Part of the reason she likes warm bread is that it produces fewer crumbs than toast. She does not like crumbs. I, on the other hand, like well-toasted toast and barely notice crumbs. You can safely assume this has led to some disagreements. Seeing her use the toaster to make warm bread drove me crazy. Well, not crazy but it did make my brain twitch around inside my head. Her brain did some twitching too. I not only eat crumby toast, I do it in bed while reading the Sunday paper—not even noticing the crumbs raining on the previously pristine sheets.

Our relationship is full of stupid little irritants like this. All relationships are. We used to try to fix each other, but that worked about as well as trying to unchew a stick of bubblegum. What has worked is taking care of ourselves and learning to accept each other—crumbs and all. Her warm bread irritates my mind, while my toast crumbs are a physical irritant to her when she climbs into bed. Although one is mental and one is physical, they are both very real. I spent time trying to convince her to use the toaster properly and eat real toast. She tried to keep my crumbs out of the bed. In the end, we realized we could not make the other do things the way we felt was "right," so we both adjusted our reactions. I stopped rolling my eyes and shivering whenever I saw her eating warm bread, and she quit groaning and flailing about whenever she encountered a crumb. We stopped the twitching by realizing that lasting love comes with irritants that you sometimes must learn to live with. (There is more to the crumb story coming up—stay tuned.)

Need Some Tips?

The rest of this chapter is devoted to tips to help improve your relationships. I'm warning you now—none of the following suggestions are magic bullets that instantly fix your problems. I don't have any secret age-old wisdom handed down from generation to generation. In fact, you probably know all this stuff already, but don't thoughtfully make use of what you know when the pressure is on. You don't move from knowing to doing. That is understandable, because in emotionally charged and stressful situations it is difficult to step back, search your memory, and control your reactions. These things can be helpful, but they take practice and thoughtfulness.

- Work at it: Relationships take effort. You have to put in *some* time and energy whether the relationship is with your sweetie or your gas station attendant. Your primary relationship should get most of your attention. Other relationships get what you can give. Since you can't change other people, most of your work should focus on what you bring to the relationship, what you can do better.

- What is obvious to you is obvious to you: A lot of relationship problems arise from lack of information (or intentional misinformation, or the wrong information). If you need something from a relationship, don't assume that your need is obvious to the other person and don't assume that your actions and words are always interpreted the way you mean them. There is always a gap between what you say and what the other person hears. Communication is all about bridging that gap.

- Practice active listening and thoughtful speaking: Be sure to be clear. This goes back to naming your needs. When you name your needs, people do not have to guess about what those needs may or may not be.

Back to the crumbs. Tasha needs to crawl into bed without feeling like she is curling up in a sandbox. She needs a bed without crumbs. I need to relax in bed on Sunday mornings with the newspaper and some toast (or, to tell the truth, on any other day of the week with some other crumbly food). We both respected each other's needs, but this put us at odds with each other until we learned to first let go of the anger and frustration that the other's needs generated. Then we had to deal with the problem. She accepted my need to veg out and munch while I watched TV. She just wanted me to clean up the crumbs that bothered her so much. I did my best, but no matter how hard I tried to de-crumb, I was not able to do it to her standard. She sees and feels crumbs my senses simply do not detect. I had another need. I needed her to realize I was, in fact, trying my best. With some letting go, some understanding, some give, and some take, we have managed to name and meet our needs. I eat in bed. I make a mess. I clean up after myself. She does her own crumb inspection and removal before she gets into bed (which I believe involves some sort of subatomic microscope and tweezers).

How you name your needs may be as important as naming them in the first place. The fact is, your needs are not going to be met if you place too much blame or demand on another person. I do my best to clean up my crumbs, but her need is not really met until she does a final crumb inspection and removal before sliding into bed.

Saying "I need you to . . ." is not the same as saying "I need . . .". Nobody else cares as much about your needs as you do. If you want others to care about your needs, you need to spell out those needs in nonaccusatory, nonblaming, nondemanding language, something along the lines of "I need _____ because _____. Can you help me by _____?" State your need clearly and also clearly ask for the assistance needed from the other party.

- Turn off technology: Cell phones, text messaging, e-mail, instant messaging, chat rooms, social networking, Web sites, and other technologies make it easier than ever to connect with other people. While these technologies can be useful, they can also get in the way of relationships. Some people spend so much time with their online "friends" that they allow important real-life relationships to suffer. These technologies also tend to be more useful for building and maintaining numerous shallow relationships than they are for developing deep and meaningful relationships. Body language and verbal nuance are hard to convey through these communication streams. I think it is wise to turn them off from time to time and focus on interacting face-to-face with real people.

- Lead with love not ego: Our big, greedy human egos get in the way sometimes, making it hard to interrelate and interpret signals from other people. It's usually unintentional, but we tend to make all situations *me*-centric: What hurts *me*? What helps *me*? How does this affect *me*? What's in it for *me*? What does this cost *me*? Where does this situation take *me*? Sometimes we need to step away from our egos and guide our decision-making with the love we feel for the other person. I have a hard time doing this as a parent. At times, I want my children to make choices that are best for *me*. I want them to make choices that make me look like a good dad, are in line with my long-term wishes for them, meet my expectations, and are convenient for me. When I catch myself having such selfish feelings, I do my best to let go of them. While my mind may be momentarily selfish, my true desire is for them to make their own choices and learn from their successes and mistakes. I'm a part of their lives, but their lives are not about me.

- Take inventory of your feelings and attitudes toward people you interact with: What we've touched on throughout the book is that you have to know yourself—

your thoughts and feelings—if you are going to keep your smile. Inventorying your mind-set about important relationships can clarify your thinking and provide valuable insight into how to best nurture and manage those relationships. Space is provided to list relationships and jot notes about your thoughts and feelings regarding them. Don't complicate this activity; just write down a name and then list the first thoughts and feelings that pop into your mind about that person. After a moment or two, move on to another person. Later, come back and review your notes, looking for connections or insights.

_____

_____

_____

_____

_____

_____

_____

_____

_____

- Don't belittle people: Don't tear people down. Period. Not in front of them. Not in front of others. Not to yourself. This may sound simple, but it is far from easy. Ripping others is an easy way to build up yourself, and we all do it more than we think. We disrespect people's attitudes and attire, outlooks and orientations, weight and wherewithal, education and elocution, religion and reputation. We pick away at their weaknesses to strengthen ourselves.

  Look closely at the last few weeks of your life and you will realize you have done these things. Maybe not a lot, maybe not intentionally, but it happens to all of us. Stepping away from this habit allows us to approach relationships more honestly and with fewer walls.

- Keep your voice down: Do you like to be yelled at? Are you more productive, thoughtful, sensitive, loving, calm, or responsive when someone growls at you? When we get upset we get loud, and whoever we are being loud at gets defensive and louder. And then we get defensive and raise the volume even more. Yelling does not fix problems. If anything, it makes them worse by aggravating already tense situations. We all know this, but we still fall into the raised-voice trap. Next time the volume starts going up, take a big breath, and start using a calmer, quieter voice. It won't be easy to do because every nerve in your body probably wants to shout back, but you can defuse tense situations with a quiet demeanor.

- Listen more than you speak: We humans like to hear ourselves talk. Sometimes we get so busy listening to ourselves share our wonderful ideas and insightful thoughts that we fail to realize nobody is really listening. Try talking to an average teenager and you quickly learn how numbing others really find your words. If I had said three more words to The Boy Zoë brought home, his head would have exploded right there in our kitchen. When we bring ourselves to stop talking and really listen to what other people are saying, we learn a lot and improve our relationships. The key here is to not just stop talking but to *really* listen.

- Timing is everything: Choosing when to have tough conversations is an art. Picking the wrong time can lead to more trouble, more chaos, and more tough conversations. The beginning of a three-hour car ride—with the kids in the backseat—for a week-long vacation at Grandma's is not a good time to start arguing about the credit card bill. The middle of a romantic dinner is not a good time to start a conversation about his thinning hair or her expanding backside. Thinking about the when and where of such conversations may not make them easier, but it can keep tough conversations from being more difficult than they have to be.

- Self-edit: Just because you think it does not mean you have to say it. I have tried hard to learn this, but I can't help it sometimes. Things pop into my head and then spray right out my mouth. It is like the don't-say-dumb-stuff filter was not installed in my brain. I am always reminding myself I do not have to say what I think the moment I think it. I have to remember people do not want or need to hear everything that pops into my head. It's okay to think whatever pops into your head, but you don't have to say it aloud. Biting your tongue might help, thinking about how your words affect whoever is listening might help, or counting to ten might help.

- Realize that *right* is not the same as *my way*: There are many right ways to do things. For example, if I have a wall to paint, I could use a brush, a roller, a spray gun, a sponge, a wad of cloth, a small mammal, or a paintball gun. I could use oil, latex, or acrylic paint. I could tape the trim or paint freehand. Any of these things could pass as *right*, but you may not agree with my choices because that is not the way *you* would go about painting a wall.

  Equating doing things *right* with doing them *my way* is about power and control. Sometimes we need that power and control, but other times having too much power and control over other people leads to problems. If you want your sweetie to fold the laundry and then gripe because he did not do it right (meaning your way), you are asking for problems. Little things such as the laundry, toothpaste, and toast may cause problems when ideas about what is right differ. You may want to stubbornly stand up for your vision of right because you know deep down in the bottom of your soul that toilet paper is supposed to unroll from the front and not the back. In some situations, it is better to give up some power and control for the sake of your relationship. If we are willing to fight for our opinions about these small things, what happens when we disagree about what is right when it comes to big things like child rearing, money handling, and religion?

At those times, it is harder to let go of your need for control and be more accepting of someone else's idea of right. Situations require open communication, give-and-take, and a clear view of the big picture. You have to know which fights are worth fighting and when you can step back and let someone else be right.

- Speak with your actions: When I tell Tasha I love her she knows it's true, because she can look back at decades of actions verifying my words. Your true self is revealed more by your actions than by your words. I can say I am going to take out the garbage, but the garbage is not out until I get off my butt and take it out. I can promise to listen better, but those words are meaningless unless I actually listen. I can chatter on and on about my plans to lose ten pounds, but those ten pounds are going to hang around my midsection until I change my eating and exercise habits. Our actions are always speaking for us. What we need to do is make sure the actions are conveying the messages we want others to receive.

- Scale down expectations: Sometimes we expect too much from the people around us. We expect three-year-olds to behave like six-year-olds. We expect teenagers to behave like adults. We expect our sweeties to behave like the young, sexy, apparently perfect men or women we see in the movies. The reality is that most of our expectations are set too high for most of the people we interact with. I'm not suggesting you do away with expectations, just that you make them more realistic.

- Keep your sense of humor: Sometimes we take life way too seriously and miss chances for fun, smiles, and laughter from ourselves. Lighten up. Look for chances to enjoy the simple humor in life. Laugh at yourself. See the silliness that is all around you.

- Keep the love alive: Find time in your life to do special things with people you love. Make date night a monthly (or weekly!) habit with your sweetie. Ensure your own children are getting the attention they need. Look for simple ways to show the people you love that you do, in fact, love them. These do not need to be grand gestures. You do not have to spend lots of money. Look for simple, heartfelt ways to show your love. Tasha and I like to go on dates to the lumberyard or garden center, leave each other short notes, and blow each other kisses. These are not big fancy things, but they do help keep us connected. If you are feeling disconnected from someone you love, look for a simple way to reconnect.

Why Doesn't He Understand?

Because 95 percent of the readers of this book are women, because I am repeatedly asked this question during training sessions about managing stress, and because we're nearing the end of a chapter on relationships, I guess it is time to write about why so many of you ask, "Why doesn't he understand?" Here are some questions and comments I have jotted down from caregivers I have met over the last few years:

- "I come home from the center, and I am just exhausted. I want to plop down on the couch and unwind next to him for a while, but as soon as I do he asks what *I* am making for dinner. I'm tired and would like him to make dinner once in a while. *Why doesn't he understand?*"

- "Sometimes when I have a bad day I need to vent and he is the only one around, so I start talking and probably crying and he just gets this confused stupid look on his face and tries to tell me how to fix my problems. *He doesn't understand* that I just need him to listen to me."

- "I do family child care for like seventy-five hours a week. On Friday nights my husband and I always go out for dinner. I love this part because I crave a glass of wine and some adult conversation, but by the time the main course arrives he's just gawking at me and raising his eyebrows. *He just doesn't understand* that I am tired and don't feel sexy at all. I love that he wants me, but I just don't have the energy."

We've learned a great deal about men in these examples. Most of us think a lot about food and sex and have no inkling how to appropriately respond to a crying woman. To your average guy, a crying woman is like kryptonite is to Superman. I am, of course, generalizing here, but I think there are valid reasons for my generalizations. I have over forty years of experience as a guy, I know lots of guys, and I have heard lots of women talk about the guys in their lives. We think about food. We think about sex. We don't know what to do when you cry.

Want to know *why* guys don't understand? It is simple: because they are guys. They think differently, they communicate differently, they have different drives, they process emotions differently, and they sure as hell don't know what to do when you cry. Oh, want to know something else? They wonder why *you* don't understand either. June Cleaver always had dinner waiting for Ward and the boys. Princess Leia never cried. And Playboy Bunnies always look like they are ready for action. *What's your problem?*

Let's face it: men don't understand women; women don't understand men. All we can hope for is to meet somewhere in the middle and muddle through. It seems to be working—the world's population is always going up. I have, however, put together some tips for men and women on how to better relate to the opposite sex.

TIPS FOR WOMEN

- Sometimes guys really don't have anything to say. It does not mean they are upset. It does not mean you did something wrong. It does not mean he did something wrong. It just means that he doesn't have anything to say. Don't push him to talk.

- One of the reasons men do communicate is to solve problems. They are wired to try to fix things. Don't be upset when he tries to solve your problems. Be happy he is trying to help, even if you don't want that help. If you need to vent, tell him that you have to get something off your chest and you do not need solutions right now, but you really do need him to listen while you let it out.

- Men usually say what they mean, and you can take their words at face value. When we are going out to eat and I tell Tasha I don't care where we eat, I really don't care.

When she says she doesn't care where we go it means something like "I don't care where we go as long as it is not one of the places you already know I don't like and as long as the restaurant you pick goes with what I decide to wear which is based on how I look in the mirror when I try things on." Take his words at face value.

- Even if it does not look like your definition of "trying," your guy is probably trying. Give him a break. I spent a few years trying to load the dishwasher the way Tasha trained me, but I would always catch her rearranging it. I could not live up to her dishwasher filling standards.

- Don't try to fix him. He is probably not broken. Remember, we cannot fix other people. We cannot make them fit our ideal of perfection; trying to change people to fit our expectations of them generally leads to trouble.

TIPS FOR MEN

- DON'T try to solve her problems—EVER—unless she asks for help. Just listen—REALLY listen—and be supportive.

- Much of the time, women communicate for the sake of communicating. It is how they bond and build connections. This means that their conversations are full of details that are missing from most male conversations. Details that you don't think you need to hear. Details that make it hard for you to follow the conversation. Listen to these small details . . . without letting your eyes glaze over. She is not trying to bore you, she is trying to share with you and become more connected to you.

- Guys are usually all about trusting facts and numbers and proof. Women are more intuitive and trusting of their feelings. Realize she is different and let her feel her feelings and trust her intuition. Don't be so ready to mistrust decisions, assumptions, and beliefs based on her feelings or intuition.

- You want to be your own man and make your own decisions, but you should also be willing to accept her influence from time to time. Look at your relationship and you probably see many ways you influence her. For a relationship to be healthy and balanced, you have to be willing to let her influence you too. You don't always have to be so stubborn; you don't always have to be right. Letting her influence some of your decisions is healthy and good for your relationship, and the fact is she probably has better taste and judgment than you do in lots of areas.

- It may be painful, but try to communicate more. Consider using polysyllabic words now and then instead of just grunting, growling, and gesturing with your chin. Talk about your day. Share a feeling or two. Sweet-talk her without ulterior motives. Make small talk. These are things that a lot of guys find uncomfortable, but women do all the time. Oh, and look her in the eyes, not the chest, when you are talking.

Tactics, Tools, and Tips

1. Body language can give you lots of clues to the people you interact with and the health of your relationships. The problem is we are often so distracted by other things that we fail to pick up on the nuances of people's body language. Our ancestors were not competing with television, radios, cell phones, and other distractions and were probably better able to see the often subtle messages conveyed through posture, facial expressions, hand gestures, and the like. Reading body language takes practice, but it might be worth the effort if you want to get better at tuning in to the people around you. Here are some basic tips:

   - Don't try to interpret solitary gestures or expressions. Instead, look for meaning in groups of movements. A person sitting with her arms crossed, ankles crossed, sunken eyebrows, and elbows resting on her knees is more likely to be upset or sad than someone displaying just one of those postures.

   - Look for connections between people's body language and their words. If their words are saying one thing and their body language is saying something else, you can be fairly sure something is wrong. If I ask Tasha, "What's wrong?" when she walks loudly across the room with a scowl burned on her face and she replies, "Nothing," I know with 100 percent certainty there is indeed *something* wrong.

- Pay attention to context. The physical setting and what is happening in that setting can also offer clues to what someone is saying with their body language. In one setting an eye roll from my wife may mean I am annoying her, but the exact same eye roll in a different setting may mean "I've been here long enough and it is your job to think of an excuse to leave and get me out of here now."

Many experienced parents and caregivers are pretty good at catching these signals from children but fail to use these same skills when dealing with the adults in their lives. Take a moment and practice. Think about the person you are in a primary relationship with and use the space provided to list some of their body language "phrases," then translate what those phrases mean to you. As you go about your day, try to pay more attention to what the people around you are saying with their bodies.

_____

_____

_____

_____

_____

2. Consider investing some time and energy in a mentoring relationship. Depending on where you are in your life, you may feel more comfortable as a mentor or a protégé. If you have a lot of experience and wisdom you are itching to share, find a protégé looking to learn. If you are in need of wisdom, seek a mentor who has the knowledge you need. You may find that your life has room for both a protégé and a mentor. These informal relationships are a great way to

share information, expand skill sets, and contribute to your profession or community. I owe a lot to mentors who have nurtured my personal and professional growth, and I have been lucky enough to pass much of their teachings on to others. Look to local provider and parent support groups as a place to begin building such relationships.

3. If you want to make any of the above tips a more prominent part of your daily life, consider creating a mantra you can repeat to help you. A mantra is a single word or short phrase repeated aloud or to yourself that helps focus the mind. Your mantra can be repeated during meditation or throughout the day when life is challenging. Examples you might want to consider using include "Really Listen," "Be Here Now," "Name My Needs," "Let Go," "Speak Kindly," "Nurture My Relationships."

   I have to admit that the first time my buddy Chris suggested using a mantra as a tool for personal growth I laughed at him. Then I tried it and found it was a useful tool for directing my thoughts and energy. The important thing is to pick the right mantra for your situation. Give it a try.

Nine

Standing Up
for Yourself

IT IS IMPORTANT THAT WE stand up for ourselves and defend our smiles. Losing your smile leaves you feeling lost, stuck, discordant, and unhappy. Your smile—and the emotional state behind it—is vital. You never fully know what kind of impact your smile has on the world around you. You never know who you may inspire. You never know how a simple interaction with you could lead someone to live their Ultimate Purpose.

Here are the words of my friend and mentor, Daphne Cole, explaining how she became a child care professional:

> When I was a teen in high school, a very dear friend of mine took me home with her one day during my junior year. When I walked into her home, her mom had several children playing in this wonderland room of music, laughter, giggling, and art! I had not thought about Mrs. McLean's home child care until I, myself, had closed my own child care home to be an involved grandmother. I did not realize what I saw in Mrs. McLean's home was the blueprint for my future.
>
> I started my early care and education career as a *babysitter*.
>
> Our family needs in 1980 dictated that I had to contribute to our household income. I worked in two shirt factories for five years. I cried every single day of those five years. I wanted to be home with our daughters. I wanted to be the one who took them to school. I wanted to be the one who saw the milestones

of their new lives. So, one day while sewing in the vents of a few thousand golf shirts, a thought came to me. Why can't I be the one taking care of my friends' children? Why can't I make a living and stay at home with our children? I usually worked through the daily company-scheduled break, because I could sew in more zippers in jeans, put more buttons on shirts, and vent more shirts, which meant I would be bringing home more money. But on that memorable day, I took my first-ever break and went around to all of my young colleagues and asked them how much they paid for babysitting services. Most everyone was paying twenty dollars a week. I went back to my sewing machine and tried to figure out how many children I would need to "take in" to make the same amount of money as I was bringing home by sitting behind the sewing machine. It didn't take me long to come up with my figures. During my afternoon break, I went back to my peers and asked them if they would bring their children to me if I opened a day care. I sweetened the pot by telling them I would cut their child care fee down to fifteen dollars a week.

I was an unregulated caregiver for six years. I got my first license in 1986 after being turned into the Department of Human Services (DHS) for taking care of more than four non-related children. This was truly a great blessing in my life, even though at the time it didn't feel that way! After becoming licensed, I found a whole new sense of what I would do with my life! My job wasn't just about caring for our three daughters, it was the beginning of a journey God had long prepared for me to live. That moment in time was the beginning of a career to not only take care of children but to empower child care providers/caregivers to be passionate and committed to all of our children.

Daphne is now director of TOPSTAR (Tennessee Outstanding Providers Supported Through Available Resources), which is a state-funded peer mentoring program for family child care providers across Tennessee. She grew from a babysitter to an early care and education professional. Over the years she organized and joined support groups, became a trainer, served as a board member of the NAFCC, created mentoring programs, and accomplished lots of other things she never would have imagined back when she was a "babysitter." Her hard work, passion, bubbly personality, and radiant smile have influenced caregivers and policy makers around the United States.

I first saw Daphne's smile in an e-mail. I stumbled upon her e-mail address on a Web site when Tasha and I were transitioning from center-based to family child care. I e-mailed her for advice. The return e-mail I received from her was full of wisdom, help, warmth, and kindness. Her smile and passion were evident in every word. She helped guide the birth of our family child care program and has been a friend and mentor ever since. Daphne's impact, and the impact of her radiant smile, has influenced others as well.

Here is what Patty Kelly, a family child care provider in Tennessee, has to say about Daphne:

> She is my mentor. Without Daphne I know for a fact that I would not still be in family child care. She has taught me to roll with the punches. She is the most honest, caring, and levelheaded person I know. She is totally dedicated to Tennessee's children and the family child care community. She is the reason we have a state conference, regional conferences, and the TOPSTAR Mentoring Program. Daphne has been instrumental in bringing family child care to the forefront as a profession.

Daphne went home from school one day with a friend and stumbled upon Mrs. McLean's "wonderland" of a family child care program. Years later, she grew from "babysitter" to professional caregiver to state program head. Her passion inspired (and continues to inspire) others throughout Tennessee and well beyond its borders. What's more, many of the people Daphne lifts up with her smile go on to share *their* passion with others. For example, Daphne inspired Patty, and in turn, Patty has inspired many other caregivers, including her own daughter. If you sat down with a pen and map and charted all the people Daphne has inspired and then all the people they have inspired, you would end up with a map spider-webbed with lines all leading back to her little corner of Tennessee. Daphne's unending surplus of passion, dedication, and smiles has led her to influence thousands of lives. My mentor Chris had the same impact during his too-short life.

Daphne and Chris are wonderful examples of what happens when you maintain and share your smile, but they are not wonders. They are not superhuman. They are not blessed with special abilities or skills the rest of us are lacking. They are not perfect nor would they claim to be. They are simply average people living their Ultimate Purposes. They have bad days, they deal with hardships, and they often struggle to make good choices. What they do that many of us don't do is manage to navigate the tough times with a smile, a positive outlook, and a firm grasp on their own well-being. They act thoughtfully, march toward their goals, and don't let the hardships drag them down.

People like Daphne and Chris can make keeping your smile and living with joy, love, and intention look easy, but it certainly is not. They would both tell you it takes commitment, effort, and drive. They would tell you that they struggle. They would also tell you that if they can do it, so can you. If you want to maintain your smile and live your Ultimate Purpose you can if you commit yourself to the task and take control of your life.

Many caregivers I have met—heck, most people—don't feel like they have much control over their own lives. If you have worked your way through the pages of this book, I hope you have gained some understanding of what you are doing right, how you can nurture yourself, and where and why you are lacking control in specific areas of your life. I also hope that you are ready to commit to taking control and maintaining your smile for the long haul.

This, of course, brings us to Steve Martin. I remember seeing him on *Saturday Night Live* back in the late 1970s. I was nine or ten at the time. I had heard funny before, but not his kind of funny. There was a big difference between Steve Martin funny and the *Gilligan's Island* funny I was used to. I had to hear more. I saved my money and purchased his album *A Wild and Crazy Guy.* I would play it over and over again in my room, marveling at its silliness, Martin's timing, his delivery, his intonations, and the fun he had with language. One of my favorite parts of the album was a short bit about Cat Juggling. Martin talks about how cat juggling has become a popular activity in Mexico, about how they take little kittens and juggle them for money, about how the kittens go "meooow . . . meooow . . . meooow" as they fly through the air. The same bit appeared in his 1979 movie *The Jerk*.

Anyway, I was listening to an MP3 version of *A Wild and Crazy Guy* the other day and realized that caregivers are a lot like those poor little kittens. We feel like we have no control over what is happening to us, that we are just going around in circles, dizzy and disoriented from it all. Then again, maybe we are the jugglers, trying to keep all these pieces in motion without dropping them or getting our eyes scratched out. If you feel like a cute little ten-week-old kitten being repeatedly tossed through the air or if you feel like the cat juggler trying to keep all your kittens in the air without losing any blood, you are the only one capable of changing your situation.

The responsibility for making any changes you may want in your life rests solely on your shoulders. No one else is going to come along and do it for you. You are responsible for your own happiness. You have to step up and take control of your life, making the changes you need to live your Ultimate Purpose. Knowing your own mind and following where your intuition leads is very empowering, but for this to happen, you have to be willing to take control.

Can You See Beyond Your Four Walls and Roof?

We often feel caged in by our own life, isolated from our dreams and goals. We become stuck in our ruts and bad habits, and then end up cut off from the lives we would rather be living. The confinement is grating and rubs nerves raw. The walls close in on us like they did when that feisty band of rebels found themselves stuck in the Death Star's trash compactor. Unlike Luke and his friends, you probably don't have a droid with access to the main computer ready to stop the walls before you are crushed. You have to stop the walls yourself.

If you manage to stop the walls from moving in on you, your next task is to stick your head out and see what the world is like beyond your self-imposed confinement. For some of us this is a very scary proposal. We feel like one of those moles in a whack-a-mole game, just waiting for a bonk on the head with a giant hammer. The bouncy carnival music plays on as we are continually whacked back down into our little hole.

You can't continue to live this way if you want to keep your smile. You need to become a Jedi Mole. I know I am messing with a couple different metaphors here, but you need to tune in to your inner self and use the force of your own mind to gain control of your life. You need to find your own way out when the walls start closing in on you. You need to grab your light saber and slash your way out of the whack-a-mole game you are stuck in before the hammer comes down again.

We've touched on some of these things before, but I think it is important for you to consider the following as you move forward in maintaining your smile, joy, drive, and passion for life and caregiving:

What three things make it hardest for you to take control of your own destiny?

_____

_____

_____

What new habits do you need to form to have more control over your life?

_____

_____

_____

Which three people can you most rely on to assist you in your journey forward?

_____

_____

_____

Which three people make it hard for you to feel in control of your life?

_____

_____

_____

What three things can you do for yourself to help maintain your focus, clarity, and control?

_____

_____

_____

Does It Taste Like Cotton Candy?

I don't just want you to take control of your life; I want you to feel primed for success. As you move forward in your life, I want there to be regular moments when you feel every cell in your body vibrating in anticipation of your next step forward. I want you to feel your potential with all your senses. What does it look like? Does it taste like cotton candy, lobster, or prime rib? What is the sound of your own personal success when you close your eyes and listen? Does success smell like lilacs or the beach at sunrise or a walk in a primeval forest? How does your success feel on your skin? Is it warm or cool or cashmere soft?

The clearer and more real you make your success in your mind the more apt you are to make the changes that get you there. That immaculate image becomes a beacon shining in front of you during tough and trying times. I want you to take a few deep breaths now and imagine living a life full of smiles, joy, love, intention, and passion, then use the space on the next page to sketch or write about that vision. Involve all your senses in the process. Make your drawing or description as detailed and complete as possible. When you feel off track or lost in the future, you can come back and use what you have created as a tool to refocus and find your way.

How Do You Think?

Even if you manage to become a well-trained Jedi Mole who has created a clear sensory image of happiness, your inner chatter can still throw you off track. We all play self-sabotaging audio loops in our heads from time to time. We repeat phrases to ourselves like "I am not worthy of success," "I am not smart enough to . . . ," "I am too old to . . . ," "I am stuck with . . . ," "I don't have what it takes to . . . ," and "I lack . . . ." I have met many providers and parents who let these kinds of inner messages rule their lives. They expect to be unhappy and unfulfilled and then are surprised when they get what they expect from life. I know a woman who has struggled for years to keep her family child care program in operation. Her biggest problem is self-doubt; she talks herself out of success. She talks about making changes to her program that would improve quality, getting more education, trying out new marketing ideas, and taking care of her own needs better, but never follows through because she questions her own worth and her ability to succeed. She is consumed by a negative dialogue that is always playing in her head. "I could revise my program policies, but . . . ," "I could start walking every day, but I can't because . . . ," "I could take this class, but that won't work because . . . ." She struggles to see herself as capable, valuable, and worthy of success. She could be a success.

Sometimes this self-sabotage happens consciously and sometimes it is taking place in the fog of our consciousness. Either way, it is destructive; it hinders our effort toward happiness. This stiffens us, making us more rigid and less likely to take on new challenges and flow with the opportunities life offers. It also weakens our resolve and drive to move forward, leaving us stranded in situations that are not quite what we desire.

To maintain our smiles successfully, we have to minimize the negative self-talk, which is easier said than done. Awareness is a first step. Just knowing what you are doing to sabotage yourself is a step toward stopping the process. Look at the child on the cover of this book; I promise you his mind is not filled with self-doubt, negative internal dialogue, or fear about change. He is in tune with himself and eager to take on whatever life presents. He is free, comfortable in his own skin, filled with boundless smiles, joy, and love, and intentionally trying to fully know his world. I wish you the same outlook and attitude. You are burdened with adult awareness, challenges, and responsibilities, but I know that letting go of these things as much as possible so you can live with the mind of a child is very freeing and empowering. I've spent lots of time with mobile infants and toddlers, and they do not lack self-confidence, drive, and passion. I encourage you to look to the nearest toddler for inspiration and try to weave their traits into your own life.

Use the space provided to make a list of negative thoughts you frequently find roaming the landscape of your mind. Make a note next to each item on your list about where that item came from and why you think it has power over you.

_____

_____

_____

_____

_____

_____

_____

YOU-HAUL

Field trips and errands will be easier, more enjoyable, and much less stressful with the spiffy new child transport unit my family child care buddy Lorraine Kirk in Perth, Australia, dreamed up. She feels a customized child transport unit would help maintain her smile and envisions a "very plush" one-seat car with a great sound system capable of towing a trailer with seating for seven children. The trailer will be soundproof, padded, and molded from recycled plastic. It will also have a floor drain to simplify periodic cleanings with the garden hose. Another nifty feature will be trailer seats wired to deliver a *mild* electric shock to misbehaving children with the push of a button from the driver's compartment. The vehicle will be available in a number of sporty colors and meet stringent environmental standards.

Is Your Good Dog Hungry?

One of my favorite stories Chris told was about an old man who took his granddaughter camping. They spent the day hiking, fishing, canoeing, and generally enjoying each other's company and the pristine patch of forest they were visiting. At the end of the day, they sat under a twinkling blanket of stars watching a fading campfire. The little girl, seven or eight years old, roasted marshmallows while the grandfather poked at the embers with an oak stick. After a long silence the old man spoke quietly and carefully, "You know, I have two dogs that live inside me—an evil dog and a good dog. The evil dog is always fighting with the good dog." Then he stopped talking and went back to poking at the fire.

The little girl watched him, waiting for the rest of the story. She waited patiently for a long time, then she fidgeted for what seemed to be an eternity, eager to hear the rest. Finally, she could no longer stand it and burst out, "Grandfather, Grandfather, please tell me . . . which dog wins the fight?"

He slowly looked up at her with a smile and said quietly, "My child, that depends on which one I feed the most," and then returned his gaze to the fire.

I tried not to include this story here since I have used versions of it in two other books, but I have yet to hear a story that so clearly and simply speaks about what must be done to maintain your balance for the long haul. All of us have a good dog and an evil dog living inside us. When we focus on life's hardships, stresses, dark moments, uncertainties, missteps, and shortfalls we are feeding the evil dog. When we make an effort to see the good in life—the joyful moments, the calm moments spent with people we love, the moments of focus and clarity—we are feeding the good dog. Feeding the good dog is harder, because the default setting on the human mind is to see potential dangers and focus on the negative. Seeing these things protected our ancestors from saber-toothed tigers, thunderstorms, and surprise attacks from other bands of hunter-gatherers when they cautiously climbed out of the trees and started walking upright through the African savanna so many years ago. Seeing bad things helped them escape from danger.

Feeding your good dog takes more effort than feeding your evil dog, but you can make it a habit. This is something that Daphne and Chris and so many others do with what looks like little effort. They manage to see food for their good dogs in places most of us miss. They see hardships as challenges to overcome. They see setbacks as opportunities to try new strategies. They see turmoil as a chance to grow. Take some time and think about your good dog and your evil dog:

In your life, who eats the most, your good dog or your evil dog? Why?

_____

_____

_____

What are your evil dog's favorite foods?

_____

_____

_____

What foods fill up your good dog? Do you feed it enough of these things?

_____

_____

_____

What one simple change can you make in your life to ensure your good dog gets more to eat?

_____

_____

_____

Where Are You Going from Here?

I hope you are bursting with energy and ideas for taking a more active role in the future of your smile. I'm concerned the rush of everyday life we all live with will overtake you soon after you finish reading. As a trainer, I see it all the time. People leave workshops and conferences bursting with ideas and insights they want to implement and internalize, and by the time they reach the parking lot, their phones ring, life takes over, and their good intentions fade. It's hard to change your life when you are right in the middle of it. It's hard to plan for tomorrow and next year when _right now_ consumes so much of your energy. It is hard to live in the moment when each and every moment is so over-whelming.

To help you move forward and stay on a path toward keeping a long-term, healthy smile, I have created a few simple worksheets you can use to track your successes and goals. The first is a two-page annual life assessment that you can complete once a year. It asks you to name some of your successes from the last year and plot a course for the year to come. The second is a one-page quarterly life assessment to be completed every three months. This form is a place where you can name some recent successes and break down your annual plan into smaller hunks. The final assessment is to be completed every two weeks and allows you to name your recent successes and set some short-term goals that will lead you toward setting goals on the other forms. The forms are available at the end of the book, but you can also download PDF versions from the Redleaf Press Web site, www.redleafpress.org. Type "Keeping Your Smile" in the search box and follow the links. The forms are intended to be easy to complete and not too time consuming, because I know your time is valuable. The intent is to provide some structure and direction for your ongoing efforts.

The notes you have made throughout the book are valuable. Use them. They are the result of much thinking and soul searching and make a good reference when setting goals. Just looking back at them when life gets trying is also beneficial and may help you through some rough patches. Looking back at these questions periodically is a good idea too. As your life unfolds, your answers are probably going to change, your thinking is going to evolve, and your needs are going to be different.

The Internet-based resources I mentioned in the introduction will also be useful as you move forward. I will repeat them here:

- The Explorations Early Learning Enews is an electronic newsletter containing articles and resources that goes to thousands of caregivers and parents around the world each month. Subscribe at www.explorationsearlylearning.com.

- The Explorations Early Learning Facebook page is a place where you can ask questions, get answers, and vent frustrations. Click "like" to join the discussion.

- The Keeping Your Smile blog is meant to help remind you to take care of yourself and maintain your smile. Short posts don't take up a lot of your time, but they do remind you to take a few moments each day for yourself. Check it out at http://keepingyoursmile.blogspot.com. You can even subscribe and have postings delivered directly to your inbox.

Another suggestion for supporting your long-term commitment to healthy living is to partner with another person or a small group of like-minded individuals. Your partners could be other parents or caregivers, but they don't have to be. Any person sharing similar goals will be a good partner on your journey. Having another person to nudge you along, to lean on when you are down, and to support you now and then can make a big difference. Truth be told, the person who supports you doesn't even have to be an adult.

Finally, keeping track of your thoughts, dreams, challenges, and successes is also helpful. I suggest that you invest in a notebook of some sort and make recording these things a healthy habit. Your notebook will become a private space where you can plot your course, relive past successes, and tune in to your inner self. If nothing else, just keep track of the things that go right in your life, the things that make you smile for real from the bottom of your heart, then refer to them when you need a boost.

Want to Look at the Sky?

Feeding your good dog is not easy. None of the things that help you keep your smile and live your Ultimate Purpose are easy, but you can make changes if you take charge of your life and make clear, thoughtful, intentional choices moment by moment. The longer we go without being personally responsible for our own well-being, the easier it is for our smiles to fade and the more likely it is that we miss more and more magical moments in our own lives. Years ago, before I started meditating, taking time for myself, thinking mindfully about my future, and feeding my good dog, I missed too many moments like this:

> Looking across the yard on a morning when the grass and leaves still have that fresh green tint of spring I see Annie on her back looking up at something. I walk over to her. Her bright eyes glisten with joy as they scan the sky. "Want to look at the sky?" she asks.
>
> I say, "Sure" and look up.
>
> "No, get down here," she orders, patting the grass beside her.

I lie down beside her, our heads almost touching. I can see a few cloud wisps in the calm blue sky, but the quivering baby leaves of the one-hundred-year-old locust tree that shades our play area are what catch my eye. Tens of thousands of them vibrate in the gentle breeze. Annie and I chat about nothing much—bugs, birds, mommy, books, boogers. We enjoy the moment. We have shared a lot of them over her short two-and-a-half years. She showed up at my house one morning and moved right into my heart. She's going to outgrow our program one day and move on, but the time we have spent together is going to be part of her forever. Her busy brain developed while playing, exploring, and discovering in our yard and playroom.

I feel a tickle on my ear and realize she is rubbing it with a blade of grass. I gasp in mock surprise as she tickles me again. I see a bit of devil in her angelic eyes.

"I didn't do it," she says with a giggle. I look away and she does it again . . . and again. . . and again.

We watch birds skip from branch to branch, high overhead. We chat some more. We listen to the other kids as they dig in the sandbox and play pirate in a red canoe that floats on a sea of green grass. We watch the world blossom; lilacs are about to bloom. It's time to go in for lunch, but breaking away from this moment is hard. My head is 100 percent in this moment with her. I am not thinking about paperwork or quality rating systems or bills or speaking engagements or the national debt she and the other kids will have to pay off or finishing this book. The thousands of things that pop in and out of my head every day are gone. I am just watching the sky with Annie. I whisper that it is time to go eat lunch.

She tells me "No, we're not done," and we don't move for another few minutes. Then, reluctantly, we get up and move on with our day.

I can't maintain your smile. I can't lift the weight of your world from your shoulders. I can't bring you joy or love or happiness or insight. I can't make your hurt go away. I can't lead you to live your Ultimate Purpose. I can't lessen your stress. I can't empower you to make the changes you think you need to make. I don't know how to do any of those things. What I do know is that you have the power inside you to do all these things. You are strong, capable, and already know everything you need to know. You just have to trust yourself, take ownership of your life, and make good choices moment by moment. You can do it.

Now go do it!

Appendix

Annual *Keeping Your Smile* Life Assessment

Complete this form after spending half an hour doing something that clears your head, then keep it accessible for periodic review.

List your top three successes from the last year:

1.

2.

3.

Your Ultimate Purpose

What is your Ultimate Purpose?

What one thing will you do in the next year to bring you closer to living your Ultimate Purpose?

Your Expenditures

During the last year, what things consumed most of your time, energy, and resources?

What one thing will you do to make better use of your time, energy, and resources in the year to come?

Your Mind-Set
How has your mind-set improved in the last year?

What one thing will you do to make your mind-set better in the year to come?

Your Environments
How have your physical and emotional environments changed in the last year?

What one thing will you do to make your environments better in the year to come?

Your Balance
How has your balance improved in the last year?

What one thing will you do to make your balance better in the year to come?

Your Relationships
What relationship successes have you experienced in the last year?

What one thing will you do to make your relationships better in the year to come?

Quarterly *Keeping Your Smile* Life Assessment

Complete this form after spending half an hour doing something that clears your head, then keep it accessible for periodic review.

What was your most important success in the last three months?

What one thing will you do in the next three months to bring you closer to living your Ultimate Purpose?

What one thing will you do in the next three months to improve how you spend your time, energy, and resources?

What one thing will you do in the next three months to improve your mind-set?

What one thing will you do in the next three months to improve your physical and emotional environments?

What one thing will you do in the next three months to improve your balance?

What one thing will you do in the next three months to improve a relationship?

Bi-Weekly *Keeping Your Smile* Life Assessment

Complete this form after spending half an hour doing something that clears your head, then post it so you will see it every day.

What was your most important success in the last two weeks?

What one thing will you do in the next two weeks to bring you closer to living your Ultimate Purpose?

What one thing will you do in the next two weeks to improve how you spend your time, energy, and resources?

What one thing will you do in the next two weeks to improve your mind-set?

What one thing will you do in the next two weeks to improve your physical and emotional environments?

What one thing will you do in the next two weeks to improve your balance?

What one thing will you do in the next two weeks to improve a relationship?